Children with Developmental Coordination Disorder: Strategies for Success

Children with Developmental Coordination Disorder: Strategies for Success has been co-published simultaneously as *Physical & Occupational Therapy in Pediatrics*, Volume 20, Numbers 2/3 2001.

The *Physical & Occupational Therapy in Pediatrics* Monographic "Separates"

Below is a list of "separates," which in serials librarianship means a special issue simultaneously published as a special journal issue or double-issue *and* as a "separate" hardbound monograph. (This is a format which we also call a "DocuSerial.")

"Separates" are published because specialized libraries or professionals may wish to purchase a specific thematic issue by itself in a format which can be separately cataloged and shelved, as opposed to purchasing the journal on an on-going basis. Faculty members may also more easily consider a "separate" for classroom adoption.

"Separates" are carefully classified separately with the major book jobbers so that the journal tie-in can be noted on new book order slips to avoid duplicate purchasing.

You may wish to visit Haworth's website at . . .

http://www.HaworthPress.com

. . . to search our online catalog for complete tables of contents of these separates and related publications.

You may also call 1-800-HAWORTH (outside US/Canada: 607-722-5857), or Fax 1-800-895-0582 (outside US/Canada: 607-771-0012), or e-mail at:

getinfo@haworthpressinc.com

Children with Developmental Coordination Disorder: Strategies for Success, edited by Cheryl Missiuna, PhD, OT(C) (Vol. 20, No. 2/3, 2001). *Teaches you to recognize the signs of this disorder and suggests treatment options that work. Presents comprehensive summaries of the literature and research findings that are relevant to pediatric therapists working with children who have DCD. Based on six years of systematic, cooperative research, this book demonstrates the success of a unique cognitive approach to intervention with these frustrated children.*

Family-Centred Assessment and Intervention in Pediatric Rehabilitation, edited by Mary Law, PhD (Vol. 18, No. 1, 1998). *"This publication should be read by everyone who provides services to children." (Francine Ferland, MSc, Professor, Program of Occupational Therapy, School of Rehabilitation, Université de Montréal, Québec, Canada)*

Torticollis: Differential Diagnosis, Assessment and Treatment, Surgical Management and Bracing, edited by Karen Karmel-Ross, PT, PCS, LMT (Vol. 17, No. 2, 1997). *"Provides a systematic approach to the assessment and treatment of congenital muscular torticollis as well as vital information on torticollis and its impact on the growth and development of children." (American Rehabilitation)*

Children with Prenatal Drug Exposure, edited by Lynette S. Chandler, PhD, PT, and Shelly J. Lane, PhD, OTR/L, FAOTA (Vol. 16, No. 1/2, 1996). *"The usefulness of this volume rests in its conceptual approach to the problem. . . . Of particular use to physicians, nurses, and therapists wishing to learn more about how to think about studies on the effects of drugs on infants and young children . . ." (Addiction)*

Occupational and Physical Therapy in Educational Environments, edited by Irene R. McEwen, PhD (Vol. 15, No. 2, 1995). *"Helps those involved with students with disabilities make sound decisions about services that will make a meaningful difference in the lives of these children." (American Rehabilitation)*

Concepts in Fetal Movement Research, edited by Joyce W. Sparling, PhD (Vol. 12, No. 2/3, 1993). *"A rich, multidisciplinary perspective on current research on the assessment of fetal movement. . . . Every department library should have a copy." (Finuala Murphy, MA, MEd, MCSP, Lecturer, School of Physiotherapy, Trinity College, Dublin)*

Meaning of Culture in Pediatric Rehabilitation and Health Care, edited by Suzann K. Campbell, PhD, PT, and Irma J. Wilhelm, MS, PT (Vol. 11, No. 4, 1992). *"A wealth of sensible and useful strategies to overcome the difficulties of acknowledging and understanding the way culture affects the delivery of effective health care."* (*Physiotherapy: Journal of the Chartered Society of Physiotherapy*)

Rehabilitation Technology, edited by Glenn Hedman, MEME (Vol. 10, No. 2, 1990). *"A powerful resource to the library of any member of the rehabilitation technology team."* (*ADVANCE for Occupational Therapists*)

Developing Norm-Referenced Standardized Tests, edited by Lucy Jane Miller, PhD, OTR (Vol. 9, No. 1, 1989). *"A very practical approach to test development . . . provides clear, step by step suggestions for test development."* (*Canadian Journal of Occupational Therapy*)

Augmentative Communication: Clinical Issues, edited by Susan M. Attermeier, MA, LPT (Vol. 7, No. 2, 1987). *"Highly informative, emphasizing the nontechnological, international aspects of AAC, which are critical for effective use of AAC systems."* (*Physical Therapy*)

Collaborative Research in Developmental Therapy: A Model with Studies of Learning Disabled Children, edited by Margaret A. Short-DeGraff, PhD, OTR/L, and Kenneth Ottenbacher, PhD, RPT (Supplement #1, 1996). *"Very helpful to the occupational therapist who would like to initiate a study in a clinical setting . . . An important addition to the library of occupational therapists who use sensory integration with the children they treat."* (*American Journal of Occupational Therapy*)

The High-Risk Neonate: Developmental Therapy Perspectives, edited by Jane K. Sweeney, MS, PT (Vol. 6, No. 3/4, 1987). *"Provides a comprehensive reference for physical therapy management of the high-risk neonate."* (*Physical Therapy: Journal of the American Physical Therapy Association*)

Vestibular Processing Dysfunction in Children, edited by Kenneth Ottenbacher, PhD, OTR, and Margaret A. Short-DeGraff, PhD, OTR/L (Vol. 5, No. 2/3, 1985). *"An interesting and rich resource on vestibular dysfunction. A valuable asset to a reference library and for therapists concerned with understanding difficulties of movement, development, organization, and performance."* (*Journal of the Chartered Society of Physiotherapy*)

Recreation for the Disabled Child, edited by Donna B. Bernhardt, MS, RPT, ATC (Vol. 4, No. 3, 1985). *"A fine book for a recreational specialist, this book brings together several first-rate essays dealing with disability and sport."* (*Rehabilitation Literature*)

Aquatics: A Revived Approach to Pediatric Management, edited by Faye H. Dulcy, MMSc, RPT (Vol. 3, No. 1, 1983). *"Very useful for physical therapy practitioners who work in a therapeutic or recreational progam, especially in pediatrics."* (*Physical Therapy: The Journal of the American Physical Therapy Association*)

Children with Developmental Coordination Disorder: Strategies for Success has been co-published simultaneously as *Physical & Occupational Therapy in Pediatrics*, Volume 20, Numbers 2/3 2001.

The development, preparation, and publication of this work has been undertaken with great care. However, the publisher, employees, editors, and agents of The Haworth Press and all imprints of The Haworth Press, Inc., including The Haworth Medical Press® and Pharmaceutical Products Press®, are not responsible for any errors contained herein or for consequences that may ensue from use of materials or information contained in this work. Opinions expressed by the author(s) are not necessarily those of The Haworth Press, Inc.

The Haworth Press, Inc., 10 Alice Street, Binghamton, NY 13904-1580 USA

Cover design by Thomas J. Mayshock Jr.

Library of Congress Cataloging-in-Publication Data

Children with developmental coordination disorder : strategies for success / Cheryl Missiuna, editor.
     p. cm.
    "Children with developmental coordination disorder has been co-published simultaneously as Physical & occupational therapy in pediatrics, volume 20, number 2/3 2001."
    Includes bibliographical references and index.
    ISBN 0-7890-1357-6 (alk. paper) – ISBN 0-7890-1358-4 (alk. paper)
    1. Clumsiness in children. 2. Motor abilities in children. 3. Child development. 4. Occupational therapy for children. I. Missiuna, Cheryl. II. Physical & occupational therapy in pediatrics, v. 20, number 2/3, 2001.

RJ496.M68 C48 2001
618.92'7–dc21

2001016716

Children with Developmental Coordination Disorder: Strategies for Success

Cheryl Missiuna, PhD, OT(C)
Editor

Children with Developmental Coordination Disorder: Strategies for Success has been co-published simultaneously as *Physical & Occupational Therapy in Pediatrics*, Volume 20, Numbers 2/3 2001.

The Haworth Press, Inc.
New York • London • Oxford

Indexing, Abstracting & Website/Internet Coverage

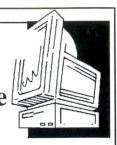

This section provides you with a list of major indexing & abstracting services. That is to say, each service began covering this periodical during the year noted in the right column. Most Websites which are listed below have indicated that they will either post, disseminate, compile, archive, cite or alert their own Website users with research-based content from this work. (This list is as current as the copyright date of this publication.)

(continued)

Special Bibliographic Notes related to special journal issues (separates) and indexing/abstracting:

- indexing/abstracting services in this list will also cover material in any "separate" that is co-published simultaneously with Haworth's special thematic journal issue or DocuSerial. Indexing/abstracting usually covers material at the article/chapter level.
- monographic co-editions are intended for either non-subscribers or libraries which intend to purchase a second copy for their circulating collections.
- monographic co-editions are reported to all jobbers/wholesalers/approval plans. The source journal is listed as the "series" to assist the prevention of duplicate purchasing in the same manner utilized for books-in-series.
- to facilitate user/access services all indexing/abstracting services are encouraged to utilize the co-indexing entry note indicated at the bottom of the first page of each article/chapter/contribution.
- this is intended to assist a library user of any reference tool (whether print, electronic, online, or CD-ROM) to locate the monographic version if the library has purchased this version but not a subscription to the source journal.
- individual articles/chapters in any Haworth publication are also available through the Haworth Document Delivery Service (HDDS).

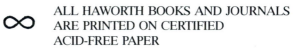

ALL HAWORTH BOOKS AND JOURNALS
ARE PRINTED ON CERTIFIED
ACID-FREE PAPER

Children with Developmental Coordination Disorder: Strategies for Success

CONTENTS

ABOUT THE EDITOR

Cheryl Missiuna, PhD, OTC, is an Assistant Professor in the School of Rehabilitation Science at McMaster University in Ontario, Canada. She is an investigator with CanChild, Centre for Childhood Disability Research, and the Developmental Coordination Disorder Research Group. Dr. Missiuna recently received a New Investigator Health Career Award from the Canadian Institutes of Health Research and the Social Sciences and Humanities Research Council of Canada that will allow her to focus on investigating the early identification of children with developmental coordination disorder, goal-setting in young children with disabilities, and cognitive approaches to intervention.

Preface

Kyle, a six year old boy, is starting to think that there is something wrong with him. He looks like everybody else, but he feels different. He has trouble doing up the button on his jeans, he can't hit a baseball, his teacher can't read his printing, and he can't tie his shoes. It seems like all the other kids in his class can do these things easily and quickly.

Kyle's parents sensed that there was something wrong with their son from the time he entered the preschool program. They noticed some subtle problems with learning daily tasks, observed a very low tolerance for frustration and have seen him become more isolated from his peers. Morning routines and mealtimes are always stressful as Kyle seems to have trouble doing simple things like spreading jam or doing up his pants on his own. Their pediatrician told them not to worry; Kyle is just a bit behind developmentally and would catch up with his peers. Kyle's parents are not convinced.

Kyle's teacher in Grade One is frustrated with him. Kyle seems to be bright enough and can tell very interesting and complex stories, but he really seems to struggle whenever he has to *do* anything. Printing, getting ready for recess, eating his lunch, arts and crafts and activities in gym class seem to be really laborious and he takes a long time to complete most tasks. She tells him to focus and to try harder, but it doesn't seem to make any difference.

Kyle more than likely has unrecognized Developmental Coordination Disorder (DCD). His story is typical and shows the anxiety, the frustration and the struggles experienced by these children, their families, and those who work with them. Fortunately, there have been great

[Haworth co-indexing entry note]: "Preface." Pollock, Nancy. Co-published simultaneously in *Physical & Occupational Therapy in Pediatrics* (The Haworth Press, Inc.) Vol. 20, No. 2/3, 2001, pp. xv-xvi; and: *Children with Developmental Coordination Disorder: Strategies for Success* (ed: Cheryl Missiuna) The Haworth Press, Inc., 2001, pp. xiii-xiv. Single or multiple copies of this article are available for a fee from The Haworth Document Delivery Service [1-800-342-9678, 9:00 a.m. - 5:00 p.m. (EST). E-mail address: getinfo@haworthpressinc.com].

xiii

strides made over the past ten years in the understanding of DCD; in identification, assessment and intervention. This book represents some of the results of a wonderful collaborative effort of researchers based in three Canadian cities. Through a focused agenda, sustained effort and teamwork, these groups have produced some of the most exciting and instructive research in the field. This volume, which brings together the results of this work, will have a powerful impact on children with DCD, their families and the therapists and educators who work with them.

I have been fortunate, due to my proximity (a shared office) to the Editor, Cheryl Missiuna, to benefit from the work that she and her colleagues have been doing over the years. This knowledge has had a profound influence on my teaching of occupational therapy students and on my clinical practice with children with DCD and their families. I am delighted that they are now ready to share this knowledge with the world.

Nancy Pollock, MSc, OT(C)
Associate Clinical Professor
School of Rehabilitation Science
Co-Investigator
CanChild Centre for Childhood Disability Research
McMaster University
Hamilton, Ontario, Canada

INTRODUCTION

Strategies for Success:
Working with Children
with Developmental Coordination Disorder

Cheryl Missiuna

Occupational and physical therapists are receiving increasing numbers of referrals for school-aged children who present with handwriting difficulties, fine and gross motor delay, clumsiness and balance problems. While in the past, some might have believed that these children did not warrant intervention, teachers today initiate referrals because they notice the extent to which children with these types of problems have difficulty participating in the classroom and on the playground. This publication is timely because we now accept that

Cheryl Missiuna, PhD, OT(C) is Assistant Professor, School of Rehabilitation Science and Co-Investigator, CanChild Centre for Childhood Disability Research, McMaster University.

Address correspondence to the author at: School of Rehabilitation Science, Institute of Applied Health Sciences, McMaster University, 1400 Main Street West, Hamilton, Ontario, Canada L8S 1C7 (E-mail: missiuna@mcmaster.ca).

[Haworth co-indexing entry note]: "Strategies for Success: Working with Children with Developmental Coordination Disorder." Missiuna, Cheryl. Co-published simultaneously in *Physical & Occupational Therapy in Pediatrics* (The Haworth Press, Inc.) Vol. 20, No. 2/3, 2001, pp. 1-4; and: *Children with Developmental Coordination Disorder: Strategies for Success* (ed: Cheryl Missiuna) The Haworth Press, Inc., 2001, pp. 1-4. Single or multiple copies of this article are available for a fee from The Haworth Document Delivery Service [1-800-342-9678, 9:00 a.m. - 5:00 p.m. (EST). E-mail address: getinfo@haworthpressinc.com].

many of the children who are experiencing academic and self-care challenges have a distinct movement skill syndrome that is recognized by the World Health Organization, and has been labelled by the American Psychiatric Association as Developmental Coordination Disorder (DCD). Although these children continue to be known by many other labels, including developmental dyspraxia, sensory integrative dysfunction, physical awkwardness, and the clumsy child syndrome, there is now an international consensus among researchers and clinicians that we will use the term DCD whenever we publish our research or clinical observations. In this way, therapists across North America and around the world will be able to access each other's literature and learn from one another.

The papers that have been compiled in this publication primarily represent the efforts of a group of researchers who have worked together for the past six years and who comprise the Developmental Coordination Disorder Research Group. Following an international consensus meeting that was held in London, Ontario in 1994, this group of individuals decided to jointly undertake a series of research studies that would help us answer a few key questions: Who are these children? What are their descriptive characteristics? What types of intervention are currently being provided? What seems to help them learn new motor skills? Based on our understanding of theory, and our observations of the children, what should work? This group of researchers, under the leadership of Dr. Helene Polatajko, has systematically developed and evaluated an innovative approach to intervention, a Cognitive Orientation to daily Occupational Performance. Contributions to this publication have also been made by colleagues from Alberta who share our interest in, and who have worked to further our understanding of, this population.

The articles in this work flow logically to illustrate the process that is followed when one undertakes the development of a new approach to intervention. First one must have a good understanding of the children who are to be served. Dewey and Wilson use the DSM-IV definition of Developmental Coordination Disorder as the organizational structure for their paper. Providing a comprehensive review of the world literature, they address the question "Who are these children?"

Once we have an idea of the characteristics of the children, therapists typically use assessments to identify and describe the problems that are experienced by any particular child. In this paper, Crawford,

Wilson and Dewey tackle the difficult process of examining the assessments that are frequently used to identify children with DCD. Their analyses indicate that two of the more common tools, the Bruininks Oseretsky Test of Motor Proficiency and the Movement Assessment Battery for Children, actually identify different children, depending upon the degree to which the children show evidence of concomitant attentional problems. These authors emphasize the importance of using clinical reasoning and multiple sources of information when identifying children with DCD.

As we move toward intervention, Mandich and colleagues outline the evidence, or lack thereof, for treatment approaches that are currently used by occupational and physical therapists in the treatment of children with DCD. Mandich argues that hierarchical models of motor development, which are the underpinnings of "bottom up" treatment approaches such as sensory integration, process-oriented treatment, and perceptual motor approaches, have little empirical research support. Newer motor learning theories suggest that learning results from the interaction of the child, the task and the environment and therapeutic interventions need to reflect that understanding.

The systematic development and evaluation of the Cognitive Orientation to daily Occupational Performance (CO-OP) is described in a three-part series of papers. The theoretical underpinnings of the approach, derived from the fields of motor learning, educational psychology, cognitive strategies and occupational therapy, provide the foundation. The series of studies that contributed to the development and refinement of CO-OP are presented next in order to illustrate the manner in which evidence has been gathered systematically to examine its efficacy. Progressing from single case studies, through systematic replication, videotape analysis, a randomized clinical trial, and retrospective chart review, Polatajko and colleagues present the results that support the use of one particular cognitive approach with children with DCD. In the final paper of the series, the protocol that has resulted from the theoretical discussions and empirical evidence is described. The objectives, key features and techniques of the Cognitive Orientation to daily Occupational Performance (CO-OP) that are believed to be important components of the approach are outlined.

Mandich's paper follows and describes, in more detail, the cognitive strategies that have been found to be useful for producing changes in motor behaviour in children with DCD. Mandich and colleagues elaborate upon the way in which a global cognitive strategy is introduced and its usage facilitated with children with DCD. Using videotape analysis, the specific strategies that appear to facilitate problem-solving and enhance skill acquisition are outlined and examples are provided.

Finally, the "Clinical Concerns" section of this volume presents a description of a small group program that has been developed and run by an occupational therapist in Alberta, Canada. Although this program developed entirely independently of CO-OP, the similarities in the two approaches are striking. Leew describes an intervention program that she designed to help children with DCD who were experiencing organizational difficulties at school. Beginning with a similar theoretical base, Leew also concludes that children benefit from learning cognitive strategies, within a problem-solving framework, and from applying them to everyday activities. Leew's program focuses solely on academic activities and does not yet have systematic research evidence, but it is a creative, and very practical, illustration of the use of a cognitive approach within pediatric therapy.

We would be remiss if we did not acknowledge and thank the many graduate and undergraduate students who have contributed to this work in various ways at many points in time. We are also grateful for the support of foundations including the Edith Herman Research Fund, the Cloverleaf Charitable Foundation, the Hospital for Sick Children Foundation and the other granting agencies, acknowledged in particular studies, who have supported aspects of the work. Contributors to this publication hope that these articles will provide therapists with new suggestions and strategies for intervention that will ultimately improve task performance and school participation in children with Developmental Coordination Disorder.

Developmental Coordination Disorder: What Is It?

Deborah Dewey
Brenda N. Wilson

SUMMARY. This paper begins with a discussion of the historical basis for the concept of developmental coordination disorder (DCD). The definition of this disorder as it appears in the *Diagnostic and Statistical Manual of Mental Disorders IV* (DSM-IV) is then provided. The four diagnostic criteria proposed by the DSM-IV are used to describe the disorder. Problems associated with the assessment of DCD are discussed and suggestions for further research are identified. This is followed by a discussion of intervention approaches that can be used with children identified with DCD. *[Article copies available for a fee from The Haworth Document Delivery Service: 1-800-342-9678. E-mail address: <getinfo@ haworthpressinc.com> Website: <http://www.HaworthPress.com> © 2001 by The Haworth Press, Inc. All rights reserved.]*

KEYWORDS. DCD, identification, assessment, intervention

Deborah Dewey, PhD, CPsych, is Associate Professor, Department of Paediatrics, University of Calgary and Behavioural Research Unit, Alberta Children's Hospital Research Centre, Calgary, Alberta, Canada. Brenda N. Wilson, MS, OT(C), is Research Coordinator, Behavioural Research Unit, Alberta Children's Hospital Research Centre, Calgary, Alberta, Canada.

Address correspondence to: Deborah Dewey, Behavioural Research Unit, Alberta Children's Hospital, 1820 Richmond Road S.W., Calgary Alberta, Canada T2T 5C7.

Support for the preparation of this manuscript was provided by the Alberta Children's Hospital Foundation and the Ruth Rannie Memorial Endowment and the David and Dorothy Lam Foundation Fund.

[Haworth co-indexing entry note]: "Developmental Coordination Disorder: What Is It?" Dewey, Deborah, and Brenda N. Wilson. Co-published simultaneously in *Physical & Occupational Therapy in Pediatrics* (The Haworth Press, Inc.) Vol. 20, No. 2/3, 2001, pp. 5-27; and: *Children with Developmental Coordination Disorder: Strategies for Success* (ed: Cheryl Missiuna) The Haworth Press, Inc., 2001, pp. 5-27. Single or multiple copies of this article are available for a fee from The Haworth Document Delivery Service [1-800-342-9678, 9:00 a.m. - 5:00 p.m. (EST). E-mail address: getinfo@haworthpressinc.com].

Developmental Coordination Disorder (DCD) has been described under a variety of labels including minimal cerebral palsy, minimal brain dysfunction, clumsy child syndrome, developmental dyspraxia, sensory integrative dysfunction and mild motor problems.[1] Collier first discussed the concept of developmental motor disorder in the early 1900s. He used the term "congenital maladroitness" to describe the developmental motor problems evidenced by children.[2] By 1925, doctors and therapists in France were noting that many children with disabilities displayed motor awkwardness. They referred to this condition as "motor weakness" or "psychomotor syndrome."[3] Orton[4] identified abnormal clumsiness as one of the six most commonly occurring developmental disorders. He indicated that different types of developmental motor disorders may exist and that disorders in praxis and gnosis might result in motor skills deficits that were different from those arising from pyramidal, extrapyramidal or cerebellar dysfunction. More recently, Ayres[5] referred to the clumsiness seen in some learning disabled children as developmental dyspraxia. She defined it as a disorder of sensory integration, interfering with the ability to plan and execute skilled or non-habitual motor tasks. She said that children with dyspraxia could attain a high degree of skill in specific activities that they practised; however, these skills were very specific and did not generalize to other similar activities. Gubbay[6] described children with dyspraxia as clumsy children who display impaired performance of skilled movement despite normal intelligence and normal findings on a conventional neurological exam. Dawdy[7] questioned the idea that children needed to demonstrate normal intelligence before being diagnosed as developmentally dyspraxic. He suggested that children's motor skills should be compared to their level of cognitive development. If motor skills were significantly poorer than one would predict based on cognitive skills, dyspraxia was a possible diagnosis.

Initially, problems in motor coordination in childhood were thought to be of minor importance, typically outgrown in adolescence or adulthood. It is now recognized that children are not likely to outgrow their clumsiness.[8,9] Research suggests that the prevalence of motor disorders in children is estimated to be between 5-8% of all school-aged children.[6,10,11] Further, investigators have reported a higher prevalence in children with other developmental or learning problems.[12,13]

The academic and social impact of this chronic condition can be significant.[11,14-17]

Although the condition has had many names over the years, investigators agree that children with developmental motor disorders display deficits in motor coordination that are not due to any identifiable neurological defect.[18] They are distinguished from their typically developing peers by a pervasive slowness in the easy acquisition of everyday motor skills, in spite of normal intelligence and freedom from diagnosed neurological disorders.[19] As a result, their motor performance is significantly impaired so that daily activities at school (e.g., handwriting, participation in sporting activities, social interaction) and at home (e.g., self-care activities) are adversely affected.[20]

The above findings attest to the legitimacy of a separable disorder of movement skill acquisition, requiring etiological, diagnostic and remedial attention. Support for this stance has been provided in recent editions of the influential diagnostic manuals published by the American Psychiatric Association (APA)[10] and the World Health Organization (WHO),[21] respectively, the *Diagnostic and Statistical Manual of Mental Disorders IV* (DSM-IV) and the *International Classification of Diseases 10* (ICD-10). In the DSM-IV the relevant entry is headed "Developmental Coordination Disorder" and in the ICD-10 it is titled "Specific developmental disorder of motor function." Although these terms clearly indicated that these children experience movement problems, they had no precedent in the existing literature.

TERMINOLOGY AND DEFINITION

The research that has investigated developmental movement problems has been plagued by a lack of consensus on two fundamental issues: (1) the name of the disability and (2) the definition of the disability. The DSM-IV[10] developed an entry headed "Developmental coordination disorder." The DSM-IV defines Developmental Coordination Disorder (DCD) as "a marked impairment in the development of motor coordination (Criterion A). The diagnosis is made only if this impairment interferes with academic achievement or activities of daily living (Criterion B). The diagnosis is made if the coordination difficulties are not due to a general medical condition (e.g., cerebral palsy, hemiplegia, or muscular dystrophy) and the criteria are not met for Pervasive Developmental Disorder (Criterion C). If Mental Retardation is present, the motor difficulties are in excess of those usually associated with it (Criterion D)" (p. 53). In October 1994, an International Consensus Meeting on Children and Clumsiness was held in London, Ontario, Canada with a primary part of its agenda focused on reaching an international consensus on the definition, and most importantly, the name of the disability. At this meeting, it was agreed that the DSM-IV term Developmental Coordination Disorder (DCD) should be used as the name for this disability.[19]

The London Consensus also described DCD as a chronic and usually permanent condition characterized by impairment of motor performance that was sufficient to produce functional motor performance deficits that were not explicable by the child's age or intellect, or by other diagnosable neurological or spatial-temporal organizational problems. At this consensus meeting, there was also a call for the development of a comprehensive diagnostic process that would distinguish DCD from other conditions. Thus, there was beginning to be some consensus in the literature regarding the name of this disorder and its definition.

DIAGNOSTIC CRITERIA

In the following discussion we will use the term "Developmental Coordination Disorder" (DCD) and the DSM-IV headings to assist us in describing this condition.

Criterion A: Motor Coordination. The DSM-IV describes the range of motor difficulties that may be experienced by children with DCD. It also acknowledges that the patterns of motor difficulties displayed by children with DCD vary with age and that chronological age and general intelligence should be considered in the process of diagnosis. Recent studies, reviewed below, have been able to describe the movement skills of these children more completely.

Missiuna and Pollock[22] found that children with DCD tended to work slower, or to trade speed for accuracy. Their pencil grasp patterns were immature and the excessive pressure in their written work seemed to be related to poor control of distal movement. Other investigators have found that children with DCD are slow but not inaccurate in the process of response selection.[23,24] Smyth[25] found that these children demonstrated poor proprioceptive function, tending to rely more on visual information when both visual and proprioceptive cues were available. Smyth and Glencross[26] suggested that children with DCD were deficient in speed of processing kinesthetic information but not in speed of processing visual information. This finding was also reported by Wann,[27] who found that children with DCD performed like children who were 4 or 5 years younger, relying on vision to maintain their posture rather that integrating visual and proprioceptive information.

Some researchers have suggested that children with DCD display deficits in the timing of action.[28-32] Volman[33] found that children with DCD had more difficulty maintaining their postural stability compared to age-matched controls. He did not believe this was due to a deficit in timing control, but rather to a weak coupling between the components (i.e., visual, proprioceptive, kinesthetic) involved in dynamic motor control. Geuze and van Dellan[34] found that about half of the children they identified as DCD did not anticipate perceptual information and therefore did not profit from the cues provided. Like Volman, they suggested this deficit in motor control were related to limitations in the processing of afferent information.

Dwyer and McKenzie[35] found that children with DCD had some difficulties with visual memory and perhaps were limited in their ability to use visual rehearsal strategies. Wilson[36] also found that DCD children had difficulty using motor imagery (i.e., imagining their movements), demonstrating an impaired ability to process efferent information. Based on the above review of recent research, one can conclude that the theories concerning the nature of the motor deficit in children with DCD are as varied as the functional problems the children present.

Children with DCD form a heterogeneous group[37] and there is no typical "clumsy" child.[38] This point is illustrated by the fact that recent studies that have examined the performance of children with DCD have drawn their participants from populations referred due to significant motor problems,[37,39-41] nominated by physical education teachers[42] or by regular classroom teachers,[9,11,43-47] screened from a population of school children on the basis of a test of motor performance,[48-52] or with suspected sensory integrative dysfunction[53] or learning disabilities.[13,54-58]

Because of the heterogeneity of children with DCD, the question that arises is whether DCD is one unitary syndrome or whether identifiable subtypes of DCD exist. Studies that are intent on finding the underlying cause(s) of DCD have tended to proceed as if they were dealing with a single, unitary disorder.[24,26,28,42,56] Often these studies are based on a theory as to what underlies the motor coordination problems of children with DCD. One theory that has been suggested is that motor coordination problems are due to an impairment of sensory integration.[53,59] It has also been suggested that deficits in visual perception[6,11,37,41,58,60-62] or deficits in kinesthetic perception[62-65] underlie poor motor coordination. Although all of the above studies have shown that children with DCD differ from non-DCD control children on a number of abilities, none of these studies has provided us with any clear evidence as to whether DCD is a unitary disorder or whether identifiable subtypes of DCD exist. This can only be done by investigating the various differences exhibited within the population of children diagnosed with DCD.

Criterion B: Academic Achievement or Activities of Daily Living. Criterion B states that "the diagnosis is made only if this impairment significantly interferes with academic achievement or activities of daily living" (p. 53).[10] Academic achievement and activities of daily living represent two distinct functional issues and should be examined independently of each other.

Many studies have found that being "clumsy" in the early years carries with it an increased risk of other learning difficulties later.[66-68] Further, a number of investigations have reported a relationship between DCD and academic performance.[9,13,14,38,52,69] These studies have found that children who display DCD perform significantly poorer on tests of academic skills (i.e., reading, spelling, mathematics) and tests of writing speed compared to normal comparison children. However, not all children with motor problems evidence learning problems.[14,44,47,70] Gubbay[70] reported that 50% of his children with dyspraxia did not show difficulties in learning. Thus, it is important to examine the academic performance of children with DCD, particularly in those areas that are primarily motor-based. Nevertheless, the absence of academic problems, by itself, is not sufficient to rule out DCD.

The second element of Criterion B is that the disturbance in motor coordination significantly interferes with activities of daily living. While some researchers have recognized that skills such as tying shoelaces and fastening buttons should be examined,[71] the impact of DCD on the performance of self-care activities has remained largely unevaluated. There are, however, some reports that provide indications of the impact of DCD on leisure, as well as the area of productivity for children–academic performance. Recent longitudinal studies of "clumsy" children have revealed that children identified with motor problems at school entry continue to display a distinct lack of coordination as teenagers.[8,9,14] Teachers' reports indicate that this lack of coordination results in difficulties in physical education, writing, handling equipment in science classes, and art and crafts. In addition, studies of children with DCD have revealed that there is an association between poor motor coordination and social-emotional problems in childhood.[9,14,17,72,73] Schoemaker and Kalverboer[17] demonstrated that even as young as six years of age, children's lack of confidence in their physical competence influences their performance of other activities. Specifically, they found that children with movement problems judged themselves to be less competent socially, and were more introverted and anxious than their well-coordinated peers. At the other end of the age spectrum, it has been found that teenagers with motor problems are very aware of their physical difficulties and that this has significant consequence for their social and emotional well being.[9,14,17,74,75] The problem in motor coordination may be accentuated further when perceptions of low physical competency result in exclusion from, withdrawal from, or avoidance of, physical activity.[76,77]

Criterion C: Medical Conditions. DSM-IV stresses that identifiable neurological disorders are exclusionary criteria for DCD. In some cases, exclusion is straightforward. Clear differential diagnosis can be made for children with seizure disorders, those with identifiable lesions, and children with muscular dystrophy. Further, at the most severe end, the diagnosis of cerebral palsy is not a problem. However, beyond this point, the process of differential diagnosis becomes more difficult. Denckla and Roeltgen[78] suggest that drawing a line between cerebral palsy and lesser disabilities of motor function and control is difficult.

It has been suggested that the presence or absence of "soft" neurological signs may provide some indication of a neurological impairment and that children who display these signs should be excluded from the diagnosis of DCD. However, there is no normative data on the occurrence of these signs in children, our knowledge about the evolution of these signs is incomplete, and we know very little about the relationship between their presence or absence and neurological development.[71] Finally, the clinical observations used by health care professionals to examine these signs are typically not administered in a standardized format or compared to age-appropriate norms; hence, the reliability and validity of these observations can be questioned. Thus, the basis for excluding children who display "soft" signs from a diagnosis of DCD is unclear.

Criterion D: Cognitive Level. According to Criterion D if Mental Retardation is present, motor difficulties must be in excess of those usually associated with it. Thus, there must be an unexpected discrepancy between the child's intellectual ability and his/her attainment. Intellectual retardation is no longer a criterion for exclusion from the diagnosis of DCD. Rather, it is the absolute difference between the child's score on the motor and intellectual test that is important. With this criterion, children with Down syndrome and Fragile X syndrome could be diagnosed with DCD. At the present time, however, most studies of DCD in children have used IQ below 70 as an exclusionary criterion.

In contrast to the reading disability literature, little attention has been paid to the IQ-motor ability discrepancy notion in the movement disorder literature. "No one has discussed the possibility that IQ may not be the most appropriate predictive variable against which any discrepancy in motor attainment might be judged . . . No attempt has been made to find out whether the motor difficulties experienced by intelligent children differ in any way from those experienced by less intellectually able children" (p. 223).[71] Further, at the present time, normative data for the entire spectrum of movement difficulties in children are not available and the research literature does not provide any indication of the appropriate discrepancy between intellectual and motor ability.

Correlational studies using motor measures as the independent variable have generally concluded that motor performance was a poor predictor of intellectual functioning, reading achievement and academic performance in children.[79-81] However, most of these studies used motor measures that were confounded by non-motor variables such as memory, visuo-motor integration, perception or cross-modal transfer.[82] Also, the motor measures were not sensitive to developmental changes over short-term intervals.[83] Wolff et al.[83] examined the relationship between "pure" motor signs and reading and language performance in normal elementary school children 5 to 7 years of age. Results showed that the children's performance on the neuromotor measures accounted for a substantial percentage of the variance in reading achievement and language performance 12 months later. Further, neuromotor status accounted for more of the variance in reading achievement than did the control variable, psychometric intelligence. These findings suggest that for children between 5 and 7 years of age there may be an association between performance on certain neuromotor tasks and performance on measures of cognitive skills. However, whether a significant discrepancy between motor and cognitive skills needs to be present for a diagnosis of DCD to be made is a question that needs further attention.

ASSOCIATED FEATURES
AND OVERLAP WITH OTHER DISORDERS

DCD shares symptoms with a number of other conditions. Awkwardness, clumsiness, or poor coordination can be indicative of DCD. However, these symptoms can also be indicative of neurological, intellectual, or sensory impairments.[18,84,85] While the descriptors are the same, the conditions are quite different.[10,38,84] Children with DCD do not show any of the hard neurological signs (i.e., clear-cut evidence of neuropathology) diagnostic of a neurological condition, and do not have any diagnosable sensory deficits.[86] Children with DCD can, however, demonstrate what has been referred to as neurological 'soft signs.' Neurological soft signs are thought to reflect subtle evidence of abnormality, not otherwise detectable.[84] Included under the designation of soft signs are such symptoms as abnormal movements, abnormal reflexes, awkwardness, associated movements, delayed motor milestones, poor coordination and general clumsiness.[84,87] However, it should be noted that one or more of these soft signs are so frequently seen in children that have no notable problems, that the significance of the presence of soft signs must be interpreted with great caution.[18,84,87]

The symptoms associated with DCD can also be found in children with learning disabilities (LD) and attention deficit/hyperactivity disorder (AD/HD) and indeed these conditions frequently share comorbidity. The level of overlap between the three conditions while not well documented is clearly greater than could be expected by chance alone. The estimates of overlap vary greatly. For example Kaplan[13] reported that 56% of children with DCD also had LD and 41% had

ADHD. Sugden and Wann[88] found 29-33% of children with LD to have coordination difficulties and Silver[89] (1992) reported that approximately 20% of children with LD had perceptual-motor problems and almost 75% had attention deficits.[90] Thus, the comorbidity of DCD LD, and AD/HD is quite significant.

DIFFICULTY IN IDENTIFYING DCD

DCD is a major public health problem for children. It is a relatively common developmental disorder with a prevalence of greater than 5% in the child population.[6,10,11] We do not, however, have a "gold" standard that can be used to identify the condition. In a recent study conducted at the Behavioural Research Unit, Alberta Children's Hospital Research Centre, we investigated whether tests of motor function consistently identified children with motor problems. The performance of the children with learning and/or attention disorders and typically developing children on the Bruininks-Oseretsky Test of Motor Proficiency (BOTMP),[91] Movement Assessment Battery for Children (M-ABC),[15] and Development Coordination Disorder Questionnaire (DCDQ)[92] was examined. It should be noted that none of these children was initially identified as displaying motor problems. We defined "impairment" on each of the above measures as follows: for the BOTMP, impairment was defined as a standard score of < 42, as recommended in the test manual[91]; for the M-ABC, a score at or below the 15th percentile was defined as impaired, as recommended by the authors[15]; for the DCDQ, impairment was defined as a score one standard deviation below the mean (M = 69.8, SD = 12.6).[92] In Table 1, the percentage of children who scored below the cutoff on each of the three motor tests is presented. These results indicated that the number of children identified as displaying motor problems differed among these three measures of motor function. We then investigated the percentages of typically developing children and children with learning and/or attention problems who met the criteria for DCD on only one, two or all three of the measures of motor function (see Table 2). Results suggested that it was not uncommon for children to score within the average range on one test of motor function, but to be impaired on others. Thus, these findings raise questions about the degree of agreement among tests of motor skills.

TABLE 1. Percentage of typically developing children and children with learning and/or attention problems who met the criteria for DCD on the BOTMP, M-ABC, and the DCDQ.

	Typically Developing Children	Children with Learning and/or Attention Problems
	n = 71	n = 27
BOTMP	11.3%	11.1%
M-ABC	18.3%	37.0%
DCDQ	5.6%	37.0%

TABLE 2. Percentage of typically developing children and children with learning and/or attention problems who met the criteria for DCD on the tests of motor coordination (i.e., BOTMP, M-ABC, DCDQ).

	Typically Developing Children	Children with Learning and/or Attention Problems
	n = 71	n = 27
Failed to meet DCD criteria on all three tests	85.9%	77.8%
Met DCD criteria on only one of the three tests	14.1%	22.2%
Met DCD criteria on two of the three tests	8.5%	14.8%
Met DCD criteria on all three tests	1.4%	3.7%

In a second study, we combined data on children identified with DCD that were collected in four different studies over a six year period at the Behavioural Research Unit, Alberta Children's Hospital Research Centre and by Dr. Helene Polatajko and the DCD Research Group, University of Western Ontario.[93] The main purpose of this study was to compare the performance of children with DCD who had been referred for occupational therapy treatment to that of children with DCD who had not been referred of occupational therapy treatment on various tests of motor skills. A second purpose was to investigate whether tests of motor function consistently identified children with motor problems.

The participants in these studies were children with motor coordination problems, some of whom also displayed comorbid learning and/or attention problems, and comparison children who had been identified as having no motor problems. For the purposes of this investigation these children were assigned the following groups. The first group included children with DCD who had been referred to occupational therapy for treatment of their motor difficulties (n = 76). Children in this group may also have had learning and/or attention problems. The second group consisted of children with DCD who also displayed comorbid reading disability (RD) and/or attention deficit/hyperactivity disorder (ADHD) who had not been referred to occupational therapy (n = 61). The third group included children with DCD who did not display RD or ADHD and who had not been referred to occupational therapy (n = 20). The fourth group was composed of comparison children who did not display any motor difficulties or attention and/learning problems (n = 155). All participants were assessed on the following measures: the BOTMP, the M-ABC *or* its predecessor, the Test of Motor Impairment (TOMI),[94] and the Developmental Test of Visual Motor Integration (VMI).[95]

Results indicated that the children with DCD who had been referred to occupational therapy and the nonreferred children with DCD and comorbid RD and/or ADHD performed similarly with scores lower than 1 SD below the mean on the VMI (see Table 3). In contrast, the nonreferred children with only DCD and the comparison children scored within normal limits. On the BOTMP, however, all three groups of children with DCD scored lower than 1 SD below the mean, whereas, the comparison children scored within or above normal limits. Overall, the performance of the comparison children on the BOTMP and the VMI was consistently above the published norms.

The performance of the four groups on the TOMI and the M-ABC was then investigated. Results indicated that the nonreferred children with DCD and comorbid RD and/or ADHD were more impaired on the M-ABC than the comparison children and the nonreferred children with only DCD (see Table 3). The children with DCD who were referred to occupational therapy displayed lower impairment scores on the TOMI than the two nonreferred groups with DCD; however, as the TOMI and the M-ABC are slightly different tests, one must be cau-

TABLE 3. Mean scores for referred children, non-referred children with and without learning and/or attention problems, and comparison children for VMI, BOTMP and M-ABC.

Test		Referred for OT (n = 76)		Nonreferred with RD and/or ADHD (n = 61)		Nonreferred without RD or ADHD (n = 20)		Comparison Children (n = 155)	
		Mean	SD	Mean	SD	Mean	SD	Mean	SD
VMI		84.3	11.4	84.4	11.3	100.1	15.4	106.3	13.5
BOTMP:	FM	31.6	11.2	40.3	12.2	48.8	9.0	59.3	7.7
	GM	33.4	11.4	35.1	7.5	36.0	6.0	54.6	7.8
	BC	29.5	12.4	35.1	9.0	39.7	4.7	57.2	7.5
M-ABC: Total Impairment Score		8.7	3.2	17.4	7.0	12.6	6.2	5.6	4.2

tious when making direct comparisons between the performance of children in the referred group and the children in the nonreferred groups.

The percentage of children who scored below the following cutoff criteria on the VMI, BOTMP and M-ABC is presented in Table 4: $\leq$ a standard score of 85 on the VMI, $\leq$ a standard score of 42 on the BOTMP, and $\leq$ the 15th percentile on the M-ABC. Consistent with first study discussed above, the results suggested that among these three measures of motor function the number of children identified as displaying motor problems differed.

The difference in the percentage of children with DCD identified by the VMI, the BOTMP and the M-ABC prompted us to examine whether these tests identified the *same* children. A significant association emerged between BOTMP and VMI scores (x^2 (1) = 41.78, $p <$ .001), with an overall agreement of 74%. The kappa value was found to be .43, which means that the agreement between these two tests (after controlling for chance) was in the fair to good range.[96] Scores on the VMI and scores on the M-ABC or TOMI were also significantly associated (x^2 (1) = 45.05, $p <$ .001), and the overall agreement was found to be 71% (kappa = .42). Similarly, there was a significant

TABLE 4. Percentage of referred children, non-referred children with and without learning and/or attention problems, and comparison children who met the criteria for DCD on the VMI, BOTMP, and M-ABC.

Test		Referred for OT	Nonreferred with RD and/or ADHD	Nonreferred without RD or ADHD	Comparison Children
		(n = 76)	(n = 61)	(n = 20)	(n = 155)
VMI		56	51	15	3
BOTMP:	FM	89	48	25	3
	GM	83	88	90	5
	BC	86	83	85	0
M-ABC Total Impairment Score		39	100	67	12

association between scores on the BOTMP and the M-ABC/TOMI (x^2 (1) = 91.81, $p < .001$), and an overall agreement of 82% (kappa = .62), which is also in the fair to good range of agreement. Thus, these results indicate that the VMI, the BOTMP and the M-ABC may not always identify the *same* children as displaying DCD.

The results of the above investigations suggest that the different measures used to assess motor impairment in children may be identifying different children. The finding that the two most popular tests of motor functioning, the M-ABC and the BOTMP, do not consistently identify the same children as displaying motor impairment suggests that we need to closely look at the characteristics of the tests. It is possible that factors such as the attention, memory or visual-motor demands of these different measures may be influencing motor performance.

INTERVENTIONS WITH CHILDREN WITH DCD

The characteristics of motor performance of children with DCD described above include slower movement time, relying more on visual than on proprioceptive information, failure to anticipate and use perceptual information to profit from cues, failure to use rehearsal strategies, and an inconsistency in motor performance not in keeping with other skilled movement. The needs of the child who experiences awkward and clumsy movement are many. Just as their motor performance is characterized by variability between children (and even within the same child), their needs are as variable. It is interesting to note that the two studies that demonstrated the most improvement in motor performance with DCD children[97,98] both incorporated an individualized approach which demonstrated that "there is no one way or best way of treating these children . . . What may be most important is that therapists keep their own visual, auditory, and tactile systems open to truly see, hear, and feel what works best for the child" (p. 792-793).[99] Who, then, is best able to identify the specific needs of each child and assist them and their families to deal with the disorder?

The one published study which examined the impact of a DCD child on their family provided an important conclusion of interest to therapists: "To pass responsibility for remediation to the school is to fail to distinguish between therapeutic intervention and educational practice" (p. 111).[75] Special education teachers, adapted physical educators and other disciplines have important contributions to make to the lives of children with DCD.[100] However, an effective approach to intervention can best be given by occupational and physical therapists who, as discussed below, are educated in the many areas of specific need in this group of children.

As the condition of DCD is so often misunderstood, being mistaken for poor motivation and effort, one of the most important needs of the children and their families is to learn and understand the concept of DCD. Stephenson's[75] study showed that, of the 31 families interviewed, thirteen believed that a problem existed before any professional concern was voiced. After living with the uncertainty prior to a diagnosis, 23 expressed relief once the difficulties had been confirmed. As Bundy[101] described, there is a need for re-framing of the problem. In an ethnographic study of thirteen occupational therapists working in a school-based practice, Case-Smith[102] identified three themes that they referred to, the first of which was "finding the key," looking beyond the outward appearance of the behavior to find why and how the problem is manifest. This is followed by sharing that information with others (educators, parents, coaches) so that people interacting with the child could have a different and better understanding of the child's behavior. This new awareness of the problem or reframing of the behavior[101] produces changes in the school and home environment, which enable the child to improve their function and, most importantly, their success. As long ago as 1975, Gubbay suggested that is was not important *what* was done, as long as something was being done to help "the clumsy child."[6] While the statement was not widely accepted at the time, it would now appear that recognition and acceptance of the problem are paramount components of intervention.

Another philosophical orientation of therapists that benefits children with DCD is that of family-centered care.[103] This promotes more involvement and collaboration with the families, as they are the constant advocates in their child's life. The critical importance of family in the life and intervention of a child has been demonstrated.[102,104] The families interviewed by Stephenson[75] were reported to single out occupational therapy as being particularly useful in providing comprehensive help, including information on services and education facilities, parent support, and liaison with school personnel. This role would be described as "coordination" by the American Physical Therapy Association,[105] or "consultation" by the Canadian Association of Occupational Therapists.[106]

A further characteristic of practice by physical and occupational therapists that promotes successful intervention is a holistic view of the child, which includes the psychological and social components of a child's life, as well as the physical component that is the presenting problem.[106] Although referrals for psychological problems are less frequent than those for functional, physical issues, therapists use strategies, which put a priority on the children's sense of themselves, their self-esteem, and their social successes.[102] Although not formally evaluated, psychological issues were very important to the therapists involved in this study. "What I value most in my work in the school is knowing that I have made a difference in somebody's life. . . . I feel that I have enabled certain students to accomplish life roles that they were not able to accomplish before. That is the most valuable aspect of my work" (p. 146).[102]

Studies of the psychosocial consequences of DCD support therapists' views of the importance of this component in a child's life. Henderson[74] found that the pattern of failing in motor performance set the stage for the development of a sense of "learned helplessness."[107] The children tended to have less of a sense of an internal locus of control, and therefore are less likely to accept the challenge and responsibility of their own behavior. Often their views of their actions and the consequences were not realistic. A physical therapy intervention that utilized an individualized approach resulted in an improvement in movement skill.[108] The improvement was thought to be related to the children's improved self-concept in relation to their physical competence and acceptance by their peers and, in turn, to an increased willingness to participate in physical activities. . . . training of physical skills only makes sense when it is accompanied by an increase in self-esteem and motivation to encounter physical activities in daily life (p. 146).[108]

There are several theoretical approaches to the treatment of children with DCD to which a physical or occupational therapist may ascribe. Whichever is chosen, an individualized approach that involves collaborating with the family, reframing the child's problems, and helping them to understand the characteristics of children with DCD, will impact upon the physical and psychosocial difficulties that the child experiences and will facilitate successful intervention.

REFERENCES

1. Missiuna C, Polatajko H. Developmental dyspraxia by any other name: Are they all just clumsy children? *Am J Occup Ther.* 1995;49:619-627.

2. Ford DR. Diseases of the nervous system in infancy, childhood and adolescence. (5th ed.). Springfield, IL: Thomas; 1966.

3. Cermak SA. Developmental dyspraxia. In: Roy EA, ed. *Neuropsychological studies of apraxia and related disorders.* Amsterdam: North Holland; 1985;225-248.

4. Orton ST. Reading, writing and speech problems in children. New York: Norton; 1937.

5. Ayres AJ. Developmental apraxia and adult onset apraxia. Torrance, CA: Sensory Integration International; 1985.

6. Gubbay SS. The clumsy child. London: W. B. Saunders; 1975.

7. Dawdy SC. Pediatric neuropsychology: Caring for the developmentally dyspraxic child. *Int J Clin Neuropsyc.* 1981;3:30-37.

8. Geuze R, Borger H. Children who are clumsy: Five years later. *Adapt Phys Act Q.* 1993;10:10-21.

9. Losse A, Henderson SA, Elliman D, Hall D, Knight E, Jongmans M. Clumsiness in children: Do they outgrow it? A 10-year follow-up study. *Dev Med Child Neurol.* 1991;33:55-68.

10. American Psychiatric Association. Diagnostic and statistical manual of mental disorders. (4th ed.). Washington: American Psychiatric Association; 1994.

11. Henderson SE, Hall D. Concomitants of clumsiness in young school children. *Dev Med Child Neurol.* 1982;24:448-460.

12. Fox MA, Lent B. Clumsy children: Primer on developmental coordination disorder. *Can Fam Physician.* 1996;42:1965-1971.

13. Kaplan BJ, Wilson BN, Dewey DM, Crawford SG. DCD may not be a discrete disorder. *Hum Movement Sci.* 1998;17:471-490.

14. Cantell MH, Smyth MM, Ahonen TP. Clumsiness in adolescence: Educational, motor and social outcomes of motor delay detected at 5 years. *Adapt Phys Act Q.* 1994;11:115-129.

15. Henderson SE, Sugden DA. Movement Assessment Battery for Children. Kent: The Psychological Corporation; 1992.

16. Kalverboer AF, de Vries HJ, van Dellen T. Social behavior in clumsy children as rated by parents and teachers. In: Kalverboer AF, ed. *Developmental Biopsychology: experimental and observational studies in children at risk.* Ann Arbor, MI: University of Michigan Press; 1990:257-269.

17. Schoemaker MM, Kalverboer AF. Social and affective problems of children who are clumsy: how early do they begin? *Adapt Phys Act Q.* 1994;11:130-140.

18. Hall DMB. The children with DCD. *Brit Med J.* 1988;296:375-376.

19. Polatajko HJ, Fox AM, Missiuna C. An international consensus on children with developmental coordination disorder. *Can J Occup Ther.* 1995;62:3-6.

20. Walton JN, Ellis E, Court SDM. Clumsy children: Developmental apraxia and agnosia. *Brain.* 1962;85:603-612.

21. World Health Organization. The ICD-10 classification of mental and behavioural disorders: Clinical descriptions and diagnostic guidelines. Geneva: World Health Organization; 1992.

22. Missiuna C, Pollock N. Beyond the norms: Need for multiple sources of data in the assessment of children. *Physical & Occupational Therapy in Pediatrics.* 1995;15:57-71.

23. Rosblad B, von Hofsten C. Repetitive goal-directed arm movements in children with developmental coordination disorders: Role of visual information. *Adapt Phys Act Q.* 1994;11:190-202.

24. van Dellen T, Geuze KH. Motor response programming in clumsy children. *Journal of Child Psychology and Psychiatry.* 1988;29:489-500.

25. Smyth MM, Mason UC. Direction of response in aiming to visual and proprioceptive targets in children with and without developmental coordination disorder. *Hum Movement Sci.* 1998;17:515-539.

26. Smyth TR, Glencross DJ. Information processing deficits in clumsy children. *Aust J Psychol.* 1986;38:13-22.

27. Wann JP, Mon-Williams M, Rushton K. Postural control and coordination disorders: The swinging room revisited. *Hum Movement Sci.* 1998;17:491-513.

28. Geuze R, Kalverboer AF. Inconsistency and adaptation in timing of clumsy children. *J Hum Movement Stud.* 1987;13:421-432.

29. Henderson L, Rose P, Henderson S. Reaction time and movement time in children with a developmental coordination disorder. *Journal of Child Psychology and Psychiatry.* 1992;33:895-905.

30. Lundy-Ekman L, Ivry R, Keele SW, Woollacott M. Timing and force control deficits in clumsy children. *J Cognitive Neurosci.* 1991;3:367-376.

31. Piek JP, Skinner RA. Timing and force control during a sequential tapping task in children with and without motor coordination problems. *Journal of the International Neuropsychological Society.* 1999;5:320-329.

32. Williams HG, Woollacott MH, Ivry R. Timing and motor control in clumsy children. *J Motor Beh*. 1992;24:165-172.

33. Volman MJM, Geuze RH. Relative phase stability of bimanual and visuomanual rhythmic coordination patterns in children with a developmental coordination disorder. *Hum Movement Sci*. 1998;17:541-572.

34. Geuze RH, Dellen VT. Auditory precue processing during a movement sequence in clumsy children. *J Hum Movement Stud*. 1990;19:11-24.

35. Dwyer C, McKenzie BE. Impairment of visual memory in children who are clumsy. *Adapt Phys Act Q*. 1994;11:179-189.

36. Wilson P. Abnormalities in the timing of imagined movement sequences in children with DCD. *DCD IV Developmental Coordination Disorder, from research to diagnostics and intervention*. Groningen the Netherlands; 1999;23-24.

37. Lord R, Hulme C. Perceptual judgements of normal and clumsy children. *Dev Med Child Neurol*. 1987;29:250-257.

38. Gordon N, McKinlay I. Helping clumsy children. New York: Churchill Livingstone; 1980.

39. Lord R, Hulme C. Kinaesthetic sensitivity of normal and clumsy children. *Dev Med Child Neurol*. 1987;29:720-725.

40. Lord R, Hulme C. Patterns of rotary pursuit performance in clumsy and normal children. *J Child Psychol Psyc*. 1988;29:691-701.

41. Lord R, Hulme C. Visual perception and drawing ability in clumsy and normal children. *Brit J Dev Psychol*. 1988;6:1-9.

42. Murphy JB, Gliner JA. Visual and motor sequencing in normal and clumsy children. *Occup Ther J Res*. 1988;8:89-103.

43. Dewey D. Praxis and sequencing skills in children with sensorimotor dysfunction. *Dev Neuropsychol*. 1991;7:197-206.

44. Dewey D, Kaplan BJ. Subtyping of developmental motor deficits. *Dev Neuropsychol*. 1994; 265-284.

45. Dewey D. Error analysis of limb and orofacial praxis in children with developmental motor deficits. *Brain Cognition*. 1993;23:203-221.

46. Dewey D, Kaplan BJ. Analysis of praxis task demands in the assessment of children with developmental motor deficits. *Dev Neuropsychol*. 1992;8:367-379.

47. Missiuna C. Motor skills acquisition in children with developmental coordination disorder. *Adapt Phys Act Q*. 1994;11:214-235.

48. Erhardt P, McKinlay IA, Bradley G. Coordination screening for children with and without moderate learning difficulties: Further experience with Gubbay's tests. *Dev Med Child Neurol*. 1987;29:666-673.

49. Gubbay SS. Clumsy children in normal schools. *Med J Australia*. 1975;1: 233-236.

50. Iloeje SO. Developmental apraxia among Nigerian children in Enugor, Nigeria. *Dev Med Child Neurol*. 1987;29:502-507.

51. Johnston O, Short H, Crawford J. Poorly coordinated children: A survey of 95 cases. *Child Care Hlth Dev*. 1987;13:361-376.

52. Roussounis SH, Gaussen TH, Stratton P. A 2-year follow-up study of children with motor coordination problems identified at school entry age. *Child Care Hlth Dev*. 1987;13:377-391.

53. Ayres AJ, Mailloux ZK, Wendler CL. Developmental dyspraxia: Is it a unitary function? *Occup Ther J Res.* 1987;7:93-110.

54. Cermak SA, Costers W, Drake C. Representational and non-representational gestures in boys with learning disabilities. *Am J Occup Ther.* 1980;34:19-26.

55. Cermak SA, Trimble H, Coryell J, Drake C. Bilateral motor coordination in adolescents with and without learning disabilities. *Physical & Occupational Therapy in Pediatrics.* 1990;10:5-18.

56. Horak FB, Shumway-Cook A, Crowe TK, Black FO. Vestibular function and motor proficiency of children with impaired hearing or with learning disability and motor impairment. *Dev Med Child Neurol.* 1988;30:64-79.

57. Lennox L, Cermak SA, Koomar J. Praxis and gesture comprehension in 4-, 5-, and 6-year-olds. *Am J Occup Ther.* 1988;42:99-104.

58. O'Brien V, Cermak SA, Murray E. The relationship between visual-perceptual motor abilities and clumsiness in children with and without learning disabilities. *Am J Occup Ther.* 1988;42:359-363.

59. Ayres JA. Sensory integration and learning disorders. Los Angeles, CA: Western Psychological Services; 1972.

60. Hulme C, Smart A, Moran G. Visual perceptual deficits in clumsy children. *Neuropsychologia.* 1982;20:475-481.

61. Hulme C, Biggerstaff A, Moran G, McKinlay I. Visual, kinaesthetic and cross-modal judgements of length by normal and clumsy children. *Dev Med Child Neurol.* 1982;24:461-471.

62. Wilson PH, McKenzie BE. Information processing deficits associated with developmental coordination disorder: A meta-analysis of research findings. *J Child Psychol and Psyc.* 1998;39:829-840.

63. Laszlo JI, Bairstow PJ, Bartrip J, Rolfe UT. Clumsiness or perceptuo-motor dysfunction? In: Colley AM, Beech JR, eds. *Cognition and action in skilled behaviour.* Amsterdam: Elsevier Science Publishers; 1988:293-309.

64. Laszlo JI, Bairstow PJ. Kinaesthsis: Its measurement training and relationship to motor control. *Q J Exp Psych.* 1983;35:411-421.

65. Bairstow PJ, Laszlo JI. Kinaesthetic sensitivity to passive movements in children and adults, and its relationship to motor development and motor control. *Dev Med Child Neurol.* 1981;23:606-616.

66. Drillien C, Drummond M. Clinics in developmental medicine, Vol.86: Developmental screening and the child with special needs: A population study of 5000 children. London: S.I.M.P. with Heinemann Medical; 1983.

67. Hadders-Algra M, Huisjes HJ, Touwen BCL. Perinatal risk factors and minor neurological dysfunction: Significance for behaviour and school achievement at nine years. *Dev Med Child Neurol.* 1988;30:482-491.

68. Silva PA, Ross B. Gross motor development and delays in development in early childhood: Assessment and significance. *J Hum Movement Stud.* 1980;6: 211-226.

69. Snow JH, Blondis T, Brady L. Motor and sensory abilities with normal and academically at-risk children. *Arch Clin Neuropsychol.* 1988;3:227-238.

70. Gubbay SS. The management of developmental apraxia. *Dev Med Child Neurol.* 1978;20:643-646.

71. Henderson SE, Barnett AL. Developmental movement disorders. In: Rispens J, Yperen TA van, Yule W, eds. *Perspectives on the classification of specific developmental disorders*. Dordrecht, Netherlands: Kluwer Academic Publishers; 1998: 209-230.

72. Smyth MM, Anderson HI. Isolation in the school playground: the role of physical competence. *DCD IV Developmental Coordination Disorder*. Groningen the Netherlands; 1999;26.

73. Wall AE, Reid G, Paton J. The syndrome of physical awkwardness. In: Reid G, ed. *Problems in movement control*. Amsterdam: Elsevier Science Publishers B.V.; 1990.

74. Henderson SE, May, D.S., Umney, M. An exploratory study of goal-setting behaviour, self-concept and locus of control in children with movement difficulties. *European Journal of Special Needs Education*. 1989;4:1-14.

75. Stephenson E, McKay C, Chesson R. The identification and treatment of motor/learning difficulties: parents' perceptions and the role of the therapist. *Child Care Hlth Dev*. 1991;17:91-113.

76. Bouffard M, Watkinson EJ, Thompson LP, Causgrove Dunn JL, Romanow SKE. A test of the activity deficit hypothesis with children with movement difficulties. *Adapt Phys Act Q*. 1996;13:61-73.

77. Hay J. Adequacy in and Predilection for Physical Activity in Children. *Clin J Sport Med*. 1992;2:192-201.

78. Denckla MB, Roeltgen DP. Disorders of motor function and control. In: Rapin I, Segalowitz SJ, eds. *Handbook of Neuropsychology, Vol. 6: Child neuropsychology*. Elsevier Science Publishers; 1992:455-476.

79. Chissom BS. A factor analytic study of the relationship of motor factors to academic criteria for first and third grade boys. *Child Dev*. 1971;35:1133-1143.

80. Rarick GL. Cognitive-motor relationships in the growing years. *Res Q*. 1980;51:174-192.

81. Symmes JS, Rapoport JL. Unexpected reading failure. *Am J Orthopsychiart*. 1972;42:82-91.

82. Neuhauser G. Methods of assessing and recording motor skills and movement patterns. *Dev Med Child Neurol*. 1975;17:369-386.

83. Wolff PH, Gunnoe C, Cohen C. Neuromotor maturation and psychological performance: A developmental study. *Dev Med Child Neurol*. 1985;27:344-354.

84. Cratty BJ. Clumsy child syndromes: Descriptions, evaluation and remediation. Chur, Switzerland: Harwood Academic Publishers; 1994.

85. Fox M. Management issues. In: Polatajko HP, Fox AM, eds. *Final report on the Conference Children and Clumsiness: A Disability in Search of Definition*. London, Ontario: International Consensus Meeting; 1995.

86. Hulme C, Lord R. Clumsy children–a review of recent research. *Child Care Hlth Dev*. 1986;12:257-269.

87. Sugden D, Keogh J. Problems in movement skill development. Columbia, SC: University of South Carolina Press; 1990.

88. Sugden DA, Wann C. Kinaesthesis and motor impairment in children with moderate learning difficulties. *Brit J Educ Psychol*. 1987;57:225-236.

89. Silver LB. The Misunderstood Child. Blue Ridge Summit: Tab Books; 1992.

90. Kavale KA, Nye C. Parameters of learning disabilities in achievement, linguistic, neuropsychological, and social/behavioral domains. *J Spec Ed.* 1985-1986; 19:443-458.

91. Bruininks RH. Bruininks-Oseretsky Test of Motor Proficiency: Examiner's Manual. Circle Pines, MN: American Guidance Service; 1978.

92. Wilson BN, Kaplan BJ, Crawford SC, Campbell A, Dewey D. Reliability and validity of a parent questionnaire on childhood motor skills. *Am J Occup Ther.* in press.

93. Wilson BN, Polatajko HJ, Mandich AD, Mcnab JJ. Standardized measures: How well do they identify children and adolescents with DCD. *World Federation of Occupational Therapy.* Montreal, Canada; 1998.

94. Stott DH, Moyes FA, Henderson SE. The Test of Motor Impairment–Henderson Revision. San Antonio, TX: The Psychological Corporation; 1984.

95. Beery KE. The Developmental Test of Visual-Motor Integration. 3rd ed. Cleveland: Modern Curriculum Press; 1989.

96. SPSS. SPSS Base 7.0 Applications Guide. Chicago: SPSS Inc.; 1996.

97. Schoemaker MM, Hijlkema MGJ, Kalverboer AF. Physiotherapy for clumsy children: An evaluation study. *Dev Med Child Neurol.* 1994; 143-155.

98. Wright HC, Sugden DA. The nature of developmental coordination disorder: Inter- and intragroup differences. *Adapt Phys Act Q.* 1996;13:357-371.

99. Willoughby C, Polatajko HJ. Motor problems in children with developmental coordination disorder: Review of the literature. *AmJ Occup Ther.* 1995; 49:787-793.

100. Sherrill C. Adapted Physical Activity, Recreation and Sport: Crossdisciplinary and Lifespan. 5th ed. Boston: McGraw-Hill; 1998; 706.

101. Fisher AG, Murray EA, Bundy AC. Sensory Integration: theory and practice. Philadelphia: F.A. Davis Co.; 1991.

102. Case-Smith J. Variables related to successful school-based practice. *Occup Ther J Res.* 1997;17:133-153.

103. Kembhavi G. A new philosophy of service delivery: The emergence of family-centered care. *Rehab & Community Care Management.* 1998;Fall 1998:34-37.

104. Pollock N, Stewart D. Occupational performance needs of school-aged children with physical disabilities in the community. *Physical & Occupational Therapy in Pediatrics.* 1998;18:55-68.

105. Association APT. Guide to Physical Therapy Practice. *Phys Ther.* 1997;77.

106. Townsend E, Stanton S, Law M, et al. Enabling occupation; An occupational therapy perspective. Ottawa, Ontario: Canadian Association of Occupational Therapists; 1997; 210.

107. Seligman MEP. Helplessness: On depression, development, and death. San Francisco: Freeman; 1975.

108. Shoemaker MM. Short and long term effects of physiotherapy for children with a developmental coordination disorder. In: Rink ME, Los RC et al., eds. *The limits of orthopedogogy: changing properties (part 2)*; 1994.

109. Missiuna C, Malloy-Miller T, Mandich A. Keeping Current in Cognitive, or "Top Down," Approaches to Intervention. Hamilton, Ontario: Neurodevelopmental Clinical Research Unit, McMaster University; 1997:1-6.

110. Polatajko HJ, Kaplan BJ, Wilson BN. Sensory Integration Treatment for Children with Learning Disabilities: Its Status 20 Years Later. *Occupational Therapy Journal of Research*. 1992;12:323-341.

111. Polatajko HJ. Developmental Coordination Disorder (DCD) alias THE CLUMSY CHILD. In: Willems GW, K., ed. *A Neurodevelopmental Approach to Specific Learning Disorders: The Clinical Nature of the Problem*: MacKeith; 1998.

112. Missiuna C, Malloy-Miller T, Mandich A. Mediational techniques: origins and application to occupational therapy in paediatrics. *Canadian Journal of Occupational Therapy*. 1998;65:202-209.

113. Henderson S, Sugden D. The cognitive-motor approach to intervention. In: Henderson S, Sugden D, eds. *Movement Assessment Battery for Children*: The Psychological Corporation; 1992:127-140.

114. Goodgold-Edwards SA, Cermak SA. Integrating motor control and motor learning concepts with neuropsychological perspectives on apraxia and developmental dyspraxia. *The American Journal of Occupational Therapy*. 1990;44:431-439.

115. Goodgold-Edwards SA. Motor learning as it relates to the development of skilled motor behavior: A review of the literature. *Physical & Occupational Therapy in Pediatrics*. 1985;4:5-18.

116. Wall AE, McClements J, Bouffard M, Findlay H, Taylor MJ. A knowledge-based approach to motor development: Implications for the physically awkward. *Adapted Physical Activity Quarterly*. 1985;2:21-42.

117. Polatajko HJ, Miller LT, Missiuna C, Mandich AD. A pilot trial of a cognitive treatment for children with developmental coordination disorder. *DCD IV Developmental Coordination Disorder*. Groningen the Netherlands; 1999:29-30.

Identifying
Developmental Coordination Disorder:
Consistency Between Tests

Susan G. Crawford
Brenda N. Wilson
Deborah Dewey

SUMMARY. In the absence of a gold standard to identify the presence of developmental coordination disorder in children, it is useful to examine the consistency of different tests used in physical and occupational therapy. This study examined three measures of motor skills to determine whether they consistently identified the same children. In total, 379 children participated in this study. The final matched samples consisted of 202 children ranging in age from 8 to 17 years: 101 met criteria for DCD and 101 children did not show any evidence of DCD. The results indicated that the overall agreement between the Bruininks Oseretsky Test of Motor Proficiency (BOT), the Movement Assessment Battery for Children (M-ABC) and the Developmental Coordination Disorder Questionnaire (DCDQ) was less than 80%. The difference in structure and style of administration between the BOT and the M-ABC appears to contribute to their tendency to identify different children. This study emphasizes the need for therapists to use clinical

Susan G. Crawford, MSc, and Brenda N. Wilson, MS, OT(C) are Research Coordinators, Behavioural Research Unit, Alberta Children's Hospital. Deborah Dewey, PhD, CPsych, is affiliated with the Department of Paediatrics, University of Calgary and the Behavioural Research Unit, Alberta Children's Hospital.

Address correspondence to: Brenda N. Wilson, Behavioural Research Unit, Alberta Children's Hospital, 1820 Richmond Road S.W., Calgary, Alberta, Canada T2T 5C7 (E-mail: brenda.wilson@crha-health.ab.ca).

[Haworth co-indexing entry note]: "Identifying Developmental Coordination Disorder: Consistency Between Tests." Crawford, Susan G., Brenda N. Wilson, and Deborah Dewey. Co-published simultaneously in *Physical & Occupational Therapy in Pediatrics* (The Haworth Press, Inc.) Vol. 20, No. 2/3, 2001, pp. 29-50; and: *Children with Developmental Coordination Disorder: Strategies for Success* (ed: Cheryl Missiuna) The Haworth Press, Inc., 2001, pp. 29-50. Single or multiple copies of this article are available for a fee from The Haworth Document Delivery Service [1-800-342-9678, 9:00 a.m. - 5:00 p.m. (EST). E-mail address: getinfo@haworthpressinc.com].

reasoning to examine multiple sources of information about a child's abilities. *[Article copies available for a fee from The Haworth Document Delivery Service: 1-800-342-9678. E-mail address: <getinfo@haworthpressinc.com> Website: <http://www.HaworthPress.com> © 2001 by The Haworth Press, Inc. All rights reserved.]*

INTRODUCTION

The increasing interest in developmental coordination disorder (DCD) raises many issues for the clinician receiving referrals for the assessment and treatment of children with motor problems. Not all of the children referred to occupational and physical therapy have DCD; the functional problems they encounter may be related to a number of other components outside of the motor system, such as attention, memory and behaviour. The identification of DCD requires a comprehensive assessment that includes a valid and reliable evaluation of the child's motor skills, as measured by standardized tests. In addition, the assessment needs to include observations of how the child interacts with his/her environment and the quality of the child's movement. Missiuna and Pollock[1] demonstrated the importance of clinical observations and teacher report in the identification of children with motor problems, and recommended that therapists evaluate the consistency of data obtained from standardized tests, clinical observations, and historical and anecdotal information.

The careful evaluation of multiple sources of information is especially important in the field of DCD because there is no "gold standard," no one test or screening measure that can be used alone to confidently identify the problem. Therefore, it is necessary to evaluate the construct validity of individual tests, accumulating evidence over time to determine whether a test actually measures what it purports to measure.

Research has demonstrated that motor problems in children can be very distressing and have significant long-term consequences; studies have found that children with DCD display poor social competency, have more academic and behaviour problems, and have low self-esteem.[2-4] The lack of identification of DCD can be further debilitating over the years of a child's development, indicating a need for a consistent valid assessment approach to early identification. Thus, it is important to determine if the assessment tools and assessment methods used to identify DCD consistently distinguish affected children.

One of the most popular measures used by North America's therapists[5-7] and other professionals[8,9] to assess motor skills is the Bruininks Oseretsky Test of Motor Proficiency (BOT).[10] The BOT is designed to assess both gross and fine motor skills. The initial factor analysis identified five factors, one of which ("general motor development") accounted for 70% of the variance.[10] No fine motor factors were identified, which led Hattie and Edwards[11] to question whether the distinction between gross and fine motor items was justified. They also raised concerns about the grouping of the items into subtests, the pattern of loading subtests into the gross and fine motor areas, the existence of sex differences on many items, low item consistency, and variable test-retest reliability, especially in girls. They concluded that "the test has little value in providing dependable scores and any decisions based on the test are suspect" (p. 111).

Other investigators have also questioned the validity and reliability of the BOT. Burton and Miller[8] stated that "the most impressive aspect of the BOT is its great and sustained popularity throughout the United States and Canada" (p. 169), but they do not feel its popularity was justified. They saw the test's largest problems as the large confidence intervals within which the true score may lie and its focus on motor *abilities* rather than motor *skills*. A recent study by Wilson, Kaplan, Crawford and Dewey[12] that examined the reliability of the BOT reported that correlations between scores given by two testers were high but the percentage of disagreement between testers was very high.

An alternative test used frequently outside of North America to assess motor skills in children is the Movement Assessment Battery for Children (M-ABC).[13] The primary focus of the M-ABC is to objectively assess, identify and describe movement difficulties in children. Burton and Miller[8] believe there has not been adequate study of either the reliability or validity of the M-ABC but acknowledge that clinicians and researchers might find it useful for screening, planning intervention, and clinical exploration. Although the reliability and validity of the M-ABC has not been established, studies of the Test of Motor Impairment (TOMI),[14] the predecessor of the M-ABC (which does not differ much in content from the M-ABC), indicate that it was reliable and useful in identifying children with motor problems. Significantly higher impairment scores have been found for children with learning disabilities and for low birthweight children.[13]

Parent report, as a source of information on children's current skills and deficits, has been found to be quite sensitive, reliable, and valid.[15,16] It can provide the therapist with a qualitative but accurate assessment of the child's skills in daily life, which encompasses the principles of family-centered care.[17] The Developmental Coordination Disorder Questionnaire (DCDQ) is a newly developed measure that assesses parents' perceptions of their children's motor skills. Initial analyses indicated that internal consistency, as measured by Cronbach's coefficient, was high (alpha = .87-.88); however, no additional studies on the reliability of this questionnaire have been completed at the present time. In terms of its validity, scores on the DCDQ were found to be significantly correlated with scores on the BOT (r = .46 to .54) and the M-ABC (r = −.59). It correctly classified 68% of the total sample of children with and without DCD.[18]

Parent report measures such as the DCDQ have a number of advantages compared to standardized tests: they are less time consuming to administer, are less expensive, and allow for the investigation of children's daily living skills.[19,20] Further, judgement-based assessments, such as the DCDQ, the M-ABC Checklist and the Pediatric Evaluation Disability Inventory[21] provide a balance between objective standardized testing and subjective clinical judgement[8] and are important to be included in a comprehensive assessment.[1,22]

Previous research has investigated if the BOT and the M-ABC consistently identify the same children as displaying motor difficulties. Riggen[23] compared the last revision of the TOMI, which with minor revisions became the M-ABC, to the BOT using a sample of preschool children and found that overall agreement between impaired and nonimpaired status was 88% (kappa = .71). In all the cases in which there was a disagreement regarding impairment, the TOMI identified the child as displaying motor impairments, whereas the BOT did not. Henderson and Sugden[13] found only a moderate correlation between the *impairment* score of the M-ABC and *performance* score of the BOT (r = −0.53). Wilson[24] reported that the overall agreement between the M-ABC and the BOT was only 40% in a sample of 43 children with attention and/or reading problems. About half of her sample, who scored within normal limits on the BOT, had an impairment score on the M-ABC. Many of the children identified by the M-ABC tended to have attention disorders as well. When both the BOT and M-ABC identified children as evidencing motor problems, they tended to have attention and/or reading disorders, indicating more extensive developmental problems.

Dewey and Wilson[25] investigated the performance of children with learning and/or attention problems on the BOT, M-ABC and DCDQ, and found that it was not uncommon for these children to score within the average range on one test but be impaired on another. It was questioned whether this would occur if the sample was clinically referred, rather than identified by test scores alone. Their data was combined with that of the DCD Research Group from the University of Western Ontario to examine how well different standardized measures worked in the identification of adolescents and children with motor problems, both referred or identified by other means. Wilson, Polatajko, Mandich, and Macnab[26] reported that the TOMI/M-ABC identified more children than the BOT, especially identifying those children who had learning and attention problems in addition to DCD. These two commonly used tests did not appear to identify the *same* children. In 82% of cases, children identified as DCD on the BOT were also identified as DCD on the TOMI/M-ABC, and children identified as nonDCD on the BOT were also identified as such on the TOMI/M-ABC. Thus, these two tests had an overall agreement of 82%, but when this agreement was controlled for chance occurrence, the kappa value was .62. This would be considered a moderate degree of agreement[27] but is seen as quite low for two commonly used tests of motor skills.

Even though there is no gold standard for the assessment of motor problems in children, it is important to determine if measures of motor skills consistently identify the same children. Thus, the main purpose of the present study was to examine whether children identified as DCD or nonDCD by the BOT were consistently identified by other tests of motor skills used in physical and occupational therapy. In addition, factors that may have contributed to the agreement or lack of agreement between tests of motor skills were examined.

METHODOLOGY

Subjects

Initial Sample

Children participating in another research project about learning and attention problems[28] served as the initial sample for this study, which was approved by the Conjoint Medical Ethics Committee from the University of Calgary. A fixed ratio sampling method was employed in several special schools and clinics (e.g., every second or fifth record, depending on the size of the facility) to telephone families and invite them to participate in a study of the causes of learning and attention disorders. The control group was selected by matching every second child in the experimental group on the basis of age, sex, and neighbourhood school. In total, 379 children and their families made up the initial sample: 224 children with learning/attention problems (see criteria below), and 155 controls. All subjects were Caucasian. None of the children participating in this study had been referred due to motor or coordination problems. Informed consent was obtained from each child and the child's parent.

Final DCD Sample

In total, 104 children met criteria (defined below) for DCD, and 250 children did not (referred to hereafter as nonDCD). The remaining 25 children could not be classified as to DCD status, because they had not completed the entire assessment of motor skills. The children in the final sample ranged from 8 to 17 years of age. To control for possible biases related to the selection of the initial sample, children in the DCD group were matched by age (within one year), Attention Deficit Hyperactivity Disorder (ADHD) status, and reading disability (RD) status to children in the nonDCD group. For example, if an 8 year old child in the DCD group met diagnostic criteria for ADHD, that child was matched to an 8 year old child without DCD who also met the diagnostic criteria for ADHD. For a full description of the criteria used to classify children as ADHD and/or RD see Kaplan.[28] Three children with DCD could not be matched to children in the nonDCD group because of the distribution of ADHD/RD status between the two groups. The final sample consisted of 101 children with DCD, and 101 matched children in the nonDCD group. Table 1 shows the demographic characteristics by groups.

Test Administration

Each child in this study was assessed individually by a tester who was blind as to the child's status (i.e., learning and/or attention prob-

TABLE 1. Demographic Characteristics

Variable	DCD Group (n = 101)	NonDCD Group (n = 101)	Test Statistic
Mean Age	11.62 yrs (sd = 1.97)	11.50 yrs (sd = 2.00)	n.s.
Sex	61 males/40 females	81 males/20 females	$X^2(1) = 9.48, p < .01$
SES: Low	25.8%	22.1%	n.s.
Middle	47.3%	51.6%	
High	26.9%	26.3%	
ADHD only	14.6%	14.6%	n.s.
RD only	30.3%	30.3%	
ADHD+RD combined	29.2%	29.2%	
Mean Estimated FSIQ	98.0 (sd = 14.5)	104.1 (sd = 12.40)	$F(1,175) = 8.80,$ $p < .01$

lems versus a comparison child who was developing normally). The psychoeducational assessment and the motor skills assessment each took approximately one half day.

Measures Used for Identification

The BOT is a 46-item test, which assesses the motor functioning of children from 4.5 to 14.5 years of age. Three Composite scores are obtained: the Full Battery Composite, Gross Motor Composite and Fine Motor Composite. Each composite score is standardized with a mean of 50 and standard deviation of 10. For this study, the BOT was chosen as the test used to define DCD because it is still one of the most commonly used tests in North America. The diagnostic criteria for DCD were based on standard scores from the BOT and defined as a standard score of less than or equal to 42 (which is the suggested cutoff for impairment) on at least one of the following: the Full Battery Composite, Gross Motor Composite, and Fine Motor Composite. To meet diagnostic criterion for nonDCD, the child had to have standard scores of 43 or more on all three composite scores of the BOT.

The Movement Assessment Battery for Children (Movement ABC)[13] is a standardized test, which is designed to identify motor difficulties in children. It contains eight tasks for each of four different age groups between 4 and 12 years. The total impairment score is interpreted in terms of age-related percentile norms, with a typical cutoff score of ≤ 15th percentile.

The Developmental Coordination Questionnaire (DCDQ)[29] is a parent report measure designed to distinguish children who have motor problems (as measured by standardized tests) from children without motor problems. The suggested cutoff scores indicate the presence of DCD, suspected DCD or no DCD. In this study, an impairment score of ≤ 53 (one standard deviation below the mean) was used to indicate DCD.

Measures Used for Group Comparisons

The Southern California Motor Accuracy Test–Revised (MAC-R)[30] measures the accuracy of the visually guided use of a pen on paper, for both hands. The accuracy score can be further adjusted for the amount of time taken to complete the tracing. Standard deviation equivalents (z-scores) are available for ages 4-11 years. The time adjusted score of the dominant hand was used in this study.

The Third Revision of Beery Visual Motor Test of Integration (VMI)[31] was the edition in use at the time the study began and was therefore used throughout the study for consistency. It assesses the ability of children ages 4 to 18 to reproduce a developmental sequence of 24 geometric forms. Standard scores with a mean of 100 and standard deviation of 15 were used in the present study.

The short form of the WISC-III (Vocabulary and Block Design)[32] was administered, and full scale intelligence quotient (FSIQ) was estimated from WISC-R norms.[33] In addition, the Blishen Index[34] based on Canadian occupations was used as an indicator of socioeconomic status (SES).

Data Analysis

The data analyses were conducted in three phases. In all three phases, only those results significant at $p < .05$ and trends at $p < .10$ are reported. Phase One consisted of a series of between group comparisons involving demographic variables, ADHD/RD status, motor skills, and cognitive skills. Analysis of covariance (ANCOVA) was used to analyze continuous variables, and chi square tests of association were used to analyze categorical variables. The first phase of analyses was followed by two sets of within group comparisons, all of which employed t-tests because within group samples were considerably smaller.

Phase Two involved comparing children whose DCD status was confirmed on both the BOT and the M-ABC to children who met criteria for DCD on the BOT, but not on the M-ABC (i.e., their DCD status was not confirmed on the M-ABC). The third and final phase of analyses involved comparing children whose DCD status was confirmed on both the BOT and the DCDQ to children whose DCD status was not confirmed on the DCDQ, using the same analyses as in Phase Two.

As part of Phases Two and Three, the sensitivity and specificity of the M-ABC and the DCDQ as screening tests were calculated. The *sensitivity* of these tests refers to the percentage of children with DCD who score in the impaired range, while *specificity* refers to the percentage of children who do not have DCD who score in the "normal" range. In addition, the observed agreement between tests (Po) and the agreement corrected for by chance (kappa) were also examined. Kappa values below 0.4 were considered to be poor, those from 0.4 to 0.75 were considered to be in the fair to moderate range, and kappa values above 0.75 were in the excellent range.[27] For this study, we used a standard of 80% agreement for satisfactory concurrent validity, as has been the usual practice for motor tests.[23,35]

RESULTS

Phase One Analyses

Demographic Comparisons

Children in the two groups were compared on age, sex, and the presence of ADHD and/or RD. The two groups were also compared in terms of SES, and estimated full scale IQ (see Table 1). The matching process was successful, because no significant group differences emerged for age, or ADHD/RD status. No significant group differences were found for SES.

Children in the DCD group scored significantly lower on estimated full scale intelligence quotient (FSIQ) (see Table 1). This group difference was due to the fact that children in the nonDCD group scored slightly higher than average on FSIQ, while children in the DCD group scored in the average range. Although this difference in mean scores of 6 points is statistically significant, it is not clinically significant since both groups scored in the average range.

There were significantly more females in the DCD group (see Table 1). Sex differences in fundamental movement skills have been documented by some researchers,[36] but not by others.[35] Given this inconsistency and given the fact that the two groups also differed on FSIQ, the next set of analyses considered FSIQ as a covariate, and sex as a factor.

Comparisons on Motor Skills

The next set of between group comparisons involved various measures of motor skills. As expected, even after controlling for sex and FSIQ, the children with DCD scored significantly lower on each measure of motor skills (see Table 2), with the exception of the VMI.

Phase Two Analyses

Agreement Between Scores on the BOT and the M-ABC

The relationship between scores on the M-ABC and DCD status (based on the BOT) was examined. Because the M-ABC had been

TABLE 2. Means and Standard Deviations for Motor Skills (Unadjusted)

Variable	DCD Group (n = 101) Mean (SD)	NonDCD Group (n = 101) Mean (SD)	Test Statistic
M-ABC	13.32 (7.79)	8.16 (4.89)	$F(1,58) = 6.08$, $p < .05$
DCDQ	57.55 (12.16)	67.50 (11.28)	$F(1,115) = 7.72$, $p < .01$
MAC-R	1.53 (1.14)	2.17 (0.85)	$F(1,170) = 10.09$, $p < .01$
VMI	91.02 (13.32)	99.42 (13.68)	n.s.

added to the test battery after a number of subjects had already been assessed, only 34 children with DCD and 38 children with nonDCD had scores on the M-ABC. In total, 21 of the 34 children with DCD scored in the impaired range on the M-ABC, and 11 of the 38 children with nonDCD scored in the impaired range on the M-ABC.

Table 3 shows the agreement between scores on the BOT and the M-ABC. If the BOT was taken as the gold standard, the sensitivity of the M-ABC as a screening test was 62%, and the specificity was 71%. Overall decision agreement was 67%, which failed to meet Riggen's[23] suggested standard for agreement.

To examine the consistency of decisions regarding DCD/nonDCD status, the raw proportion of observed agreement between tests (Po) and the same agreement corrected for chance (kappa) was calculated for the Composite Scores of the BOT and the M-ABC (see Table 4). When agreement between tests was corrected for chance, agreement between the BOT Full Battery composite and the M-ABC was in the fair to moderate range.

Confirmed DCD

The profiles of children whose "diagnosis" of DCD was confirmed on both the BOT and the M-ABC (n = 21) were then compared to the profiles of children who met criteria for DCD by scoring ≤ 42 on at

TABLE 3. Number of Cases and Decision Agreement Proportions (in Parentheses) Between BOT and M-ABC in Identifying DCD and NonDCD Cases

		BOT (Cut score at $\leq$ 42 Standard Score)	
		DCD	NonDCD
M-ABC (Cut score at $\leq$ 15 percentile)	DCD	21 cases (21 of 34 = .62)	11 cases (11 of 38 = .29)
	NonDCD	13 cases (13 of 34 = .38)	27 cases (27 of 38 = .71)

Sensitivity = 62%

Specificity = 71%

TABLE 4. Agreement Among Tests for Entire Sample (n = 202) as Measured by Po (Proportion of Observed Agreement) and Kappa (Adjusted for Chance)

Test		BOT Battery Composite	BOT Gross Motor	BOT Fine Motor	M-ABC	DCDQ
BOT Battery Composite	Po	---				
	Kappa					
BOT Gross Motor	Po	0.846	---			
	Kappa	*0.673*				
BOT Fine Motor	Po	0.791	0.667	---		
	Kappa	*0.476*	*0.264*			
M-ABC	Po	0.722	0.722	0.569	---	
	Kappa	*0.416*	*0.430*	*0.073*		
DCDQ	Po	0.744	0.729	0.746	0.682	---
	Kappa	*0.441*	*0.407*	*0.287*	*0.294*	

least one of the Full Battery Composite, Gross Motor Composite, and Fine Motor Composite on the BOT, but who were not confirmed to have DCD on the M-ABC. These two subgroups did not differ on FSIQ or sex, so ANCOVAs were not required for subsequent analyses.

Figure 1 shows that children whose DCD diagnosis was confirmed by the M-ABC scored significantly lower on the VMI ($t(32) = -2.85$, $p < .01$), compared to children whose DCD status was not confirmed on the M-ABC. There was a trend for children in the confirmed group to score lower on the DCDQ ($t(18) = -1.74$, $p < .10$). Children in the confirmed DCD group were also significantly more likely to be classified as RD ($X^2(1) = 5.13$, $p < .05$).

FIGURE 1. Results of Phase Two Analyses with M-ABC

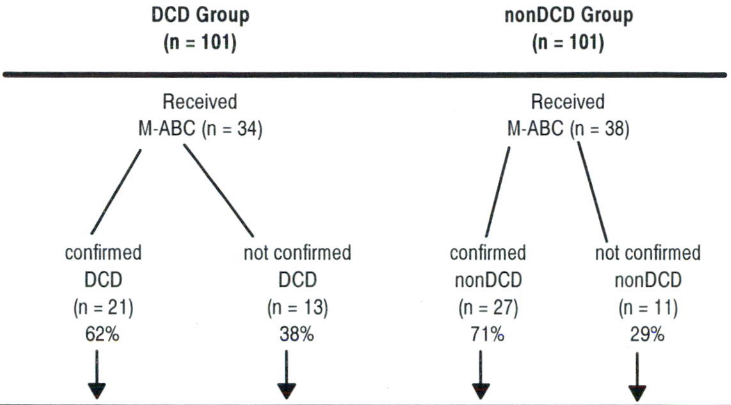

| | **DCD Group** (n = 101) | | **nonDCD Group** (n = 101) | |

Received M-ABC (n = 34) | Received M-ABC (n = 38)

| confirmed DCD (n = 21) 62% | not confirmed DCD (n = 13) 38% | confirmed nonDCD (n = 27) 71% | not confirmed nonDCD (n = 11) 29% |

	Confirmed DCD	**Not Confirmed DCD**	**Confirmed nonDCD**	**Not Confirmed nonDCD**
DCDQ	↓DCDQ	↑DCDQ	--	--
VMI	↓ VMI	↑VMI	--	--
MAC-R	--	--	--	--
RD status	↑RD	↓RD	--	--
ADHD status	--	--	--	--

↑↓ indicates a significant difference in scores in the direction shown, at the $p < .05$ level

↑↓ indicates a trend for a group difference at $p < .10$

-- indicates no significant difference

Phase Three Analyses

Agreement Between Scores on the BOT and the DCDQ

The relationship between scores on the DCDQ and DCD status based on the BOT was subsequently examined. In total, 24 children with DCD and 7 children with nonDCD scored at least one standard deviation below the mean on the DCDQ. Table 5 shows the agreement

TABLE 5. Number of Cases and Decision Agreement Proportions (in Parentheses) Between BOT and DCDQ in Identifying DCD and NonDCD Cases

		BOT(Cut score at $\leq$ 42 Standard Score)	
		DCD	NonDCD
DCDQ	DCD	24 cases	7 cases
(Cut		(24 of 64 = .38)	(7 of 70 = .10)
score	NonDCD	40 cases	63 cases
at $\leq$		(40 of 64 = .62)	(63 of 70 = .90)
53)			

Sensitivity = 38%

Specificity = 90%

between scores for the BOT and the DCDQ. If the BOT was taken as the gold standard, the sensitivity of the DCDQ as a screening test was 38%, and the specificity was 90%. Overall decision agreement was 65%, which failed to meet Riggen's[23] suggested standard for agreement. The highest agreement (kappa) corrected for chance was found between the DCDQ and the BOT Full Battery Composite (.441) and the BOT Gross Motor Composite (.407) (see Table 4).

Confirmed DCD

The profiles of children whose DCD was confirmed on both the BOT and the DCDQ (n = 24) were compared to those of children whose DCD was not confirmed by scores on the DCDQ. No significant differences emerged for FSIQ or sex, so subsequent analyses did not control for these two variables.

Children whose DCD diagnosis was confirmed by the DCDQ scored significantly lower on the M-ABC (t(17) = -2.75, p < .05) than children whose DCD status was not confirmed by the DCDQ (see Figure 2). Children whose diagnosis of DCD was confirmed by both tests were more likely to meet criteria for ADHD ($X^2(1)$ = 9.34, p < .01).

FIGURE 2. Results of Phase Three Analyses with DCDQ

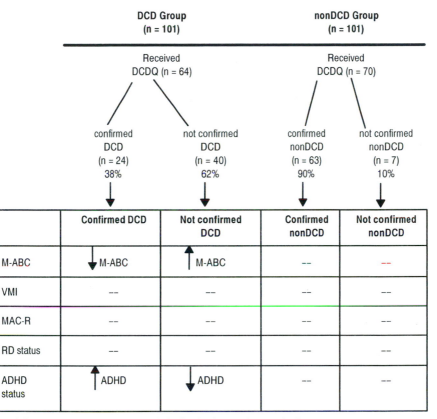

↑↓ indicates a significant difference in scores in the direction shown, at the p < .05 level

DISCUSSION

This study evaluated the consistency of test results in the identification of children with DCD. As the sample was *not* referred for problems in motor skills, comparison of these test results with functional performance and limitations to performance could not be made. The most significant findings of this study were the low levels of agreement between the BOT and M-ABC, and the BOT and DCDQ in identifying children with DCD. Over one-third of the children defined as DCD by the BOT were not identified by the M-ABC, whereas one-quarter of those categorized as nonDCD by the BOT would be classified as DCD on the M-ABC. The levels of overall agreement between the BOT, and the M-ABC and DCDQ failed to reach our criterion of 80%. Further, the kappa values were only in the fair to good range of agreement. Such lack of agreement among measures used to identify children with DCD indicates that investigations are needed that examine which characteristics of these measures may influence who is classified as having DCD. Of particular interest would be the evaluation of children who have been referred to therapy due to problems in motor skills.

The poorest agreement was seen between the Fine Motor Composite of the BOT and the M-ABC. Both the BOT and M-ABC have a predominance of gross motor items; the inclusion of a fine motor section in the BOT has been questioned,[11] and there is evidence that fine motor problems could be a distinct entity.[37] The problems associated with using the BOT to identify children with fine motor difficulties will be discussed below.

The levels of agreement found in the present study are much higher than those found in our previous research. In our previous work (see Dewey and Wilson, this volume), we also found that the M-ABC tended to identify more children with DCD than the BOT, and that children identified by the M-ABC tended to have attention problems.[26] The two studies used related subject samples but there were important differences between them. Although both samples were drawn from the same group of children who had been recruited based upon the presence of learning and attentional problems, the study reported previously in this issue simply identified children with DCD on the basis of two low scores out of five tests. The presence of reading and/or attentional problems was not controlled for in that study. In contrast, the study which is reported in this article used the same criteria for DCD, then identified the presence of RD and/or ADHD, and then found an age- , RD- and ADHD-matched child *without* DCD. The sample size, therefore, is much smaller due to the matching process; however, the possible effects of reading and/or attentional problems are controlled for by the matching process. The differences in findings between these two studies with related subject samples demonstrate the difficulty in consistently identifying children with DCD when there is no gold standard for identification.

The low levels of agreement between these tests prompted us to ask whether the differences in identification were a function of differences in the children, i.e., do different tests identify distinctly different types of children. We therefore examined how children identified, as DCD only by the BOT (not confirmed) differed from those identified by both the BOT and the M-ABC (confirmed). Our results indicated that the confirmed group had poorer performance on the VMI, a trend to poorer performance on the DCDQ, and a greater prevalence of RD.

Agreement between the BOT and the DCDQ was also examined and was found to be very high for nonDCD children but low for those with DCD. Overall agreement and agreement controlled for by chance (kappa) were quite low with similar values to those between the BOT and M-ABC. These values were much lower than those that were previously found with three different samples used in the test's development.[18] These differences may be due to the fact that in the present study the sample size was smaller, different criteria were used to define DCD and a single cut-off score was used to identify children as DCD rather than a multiple cut-off system (i.e., DCD, suspect DCD, nonDCD). However, the low agreement between the DCDQ and the BOT is not surprising. Standardized tests may be limited in their ability to identify DCD because they do not evaluate the quality of the movement.[1,38] Thus, there is a place for standardized, informal and judgment-based measures in the assessment of DCD.

Children whose scores on the BOT and DCDQ resulted in a confirmed diagnosis of DCD scored lower on the M-ABC, compared to the children whom the BOT identified but the DCDQ did not. This suggests that the DCDQ may be sensitive to identifying children with motor difficulties. The children identified by the DCDQ and the BOT were also more likely to have had attention problems, indicating that this parent report may be sensitive to those factors of motor performance that are affected by inattention. When the BOT identified a child as nonDCD, there was a high level of agreement with the DCDQ, suggesting that the DCDQ may be effective in identifying those children who are not experiencing motor problems.

When group differences between children identified as DCD and nonDCD by the BOT were investigated, children with DCD performed poorer on three out of four other tests of motor performance. The only test where DCD and nonDCD children performed the same was the VMI. The VMI is a very popular test in identifying children with fine motor and visual motor problems.[5,7] There may have been a separate subgroup of children with difficulties in the visual-motor area who were not identified by the BOT, but who would have been distinguished from children with no motor problems based on their scores on the VMI. Another possible reason that the VMI did not discriminate between DCD and nonDCD children could be because the norms are inflated, as was found by Missiuna and Pollock.[1] It would appear that the VMI norms alone are not useful as criteria for identifying DCD.

There are several important aspects of this study, which should be considered when evaluating the clinical implications of the results. As stated, the children who participated were not referred for motor problems, therefore, no comparison of test results with functional performance could be made. The present study allowed us only to evaluate the consistency of test results. Further research is needed to compare test results with functional performance. Another limitation is that the proportion of children with RD and/or ADHD in our study was larger than that seen in the North American population. This, however, may accurately reflect the clinical realities of pediatric therapists who see children with multiple learning and developmental problems as often as they see children with a distinct circumscribed problem in motor coordination. Finally, there were a larger number of girls in the DCD group than in the nonDCD, whereas, the reported population ratio is 4 to 1 boys to girls.[19,39] This may suggest that our sample *was* not a true representation of the population of children with DCD in North America, or that the prevalence of the condition of DCD for boys and girls may not yet be fully understood, or that the test used to identify DCD may differentiate by sex.[40] Further study of this area is needed.

Clinical Implications

The relatively poor consistency of the tests in identifying DCD provides pediatric therapists with information that can assist them in developing a valid and comprehensive assessment. There is some question as to whether the BOT may under-identify children with motor problems. The present study showed that the M-ABC identifies children with motor problems who are not identified by the BOT. Of particular importance to occupational therapists is the extremely poor agreement between the Fine Motor Composite of the BOT and other tests studied. The validity of using subtest scores on the BOT to identify fine motor problems in children is questioned. The use of a more global measure, such as the M-ABC, combined with clinical observations and reports on functional performance in the child's environment, may give a truer picture of the child's actual fine motor abilities.

The BOT test allows as much verbal prompting and correction as needed, which favors those children who require external controls to monitor their motor behaviour. The M-ABC is administered quite differently than the BOT, as there is more careful instruction and more opportunity for practice, but no prompting during the testing and stricter scoring criteria. It is likely, then, that the M-ABC is a more difficult test for children with attention problems. The choice of using either the M-ABC or the BOT will depend on the information already available about the child, and whether the therapist wants to "tease out" the effects of attention on motor performance.

The DCDQ is a new questionnaire that is just beginning to be used clinically. The results of this study suggest that it is most useful as a tool to screen out those children who do *not* have motor problems, as an adjunct to standardized testing. As none of the research with the DCDQ to date has been done with children who were referred for motor problems, the relationship between this test and functional performance is not clear.

In summary, this study showed that different measures of motor functioning did not consistently identify children as DCD or nonDCD. In order to identify a child with motor coordination problems, therapists should be aware of the possibility that the BOT under-identifies DCD and that the M-ABC may penalize children with attention problems. Our findings suggest that when two or more motor measure consistently identify a child with DCD, a more severe motor problem or the presence of other developmental learning problems is indicated. Information from standardized tests combined with a picture of the child's functional performance, may increase the likelihood that DCD will be accurately identified. Judgement-based assessments and observations are necessary to augment standardized tests and *to* confirm the presence of a motor problem. No one test, however, can accurately identify DCD children or replace the clinical reasoning of a therapist who examines multiple sources of information about a child's functional skills.

ACKNOWLEDGEMENTS

Many of the ideas in the paper have developed through ongoing discussion with members of the DCD Research Group, University of Western Ontario. We are particularly grateful for our work with Dr. Helene Polatajko and Angela Mandich, PhD (candidate). The Alberta Heritage Foundation for Medical Research provided financial support for travel to Calgary by Dr. Polatajko. Support for this research was also provided by grants from the Alberta Mental Health Research Fund, the Ruth Rannie Memorial Endowment, and the David and Dorothy Lam Foundation Fund. We are also grateful to the Alberta Children's Hospital Foundation for their continued support of research related to motor problems in children.

REFERENCES

1. Missiuna C, Pollock N. Beyond the norms: Need for multiple sources of data in the assessment of children. *Phys Occup Ther Pediatr.* 1995;15:57-71.

2. Losse A, Henderson SA, Elliman D, Hall D, Knight E, Jongmans M. Clumsiness in children: Do they outgrow it? A 10-year follow-up study. *Dev Med Child Neurol.* 1991;33:55-68.

3. Cantell MH, Smyth MM, Ahonen TP. Clumsiness in adolescence: Educational, motor and social outcomes of motor delay detected at 5 years. *Adapt Phys Act Q.* 1994;11:115-129.

4. Geuze R, Borger H. Children who are clumsy: Five years later. *Adapt Phys Act Q.* 1993;10:10-21.

5. Crowe TK. Pediatric assessments: A survey of their use by occupational therapists in northwestern school systems. *The Occupational Therapy Journal of Research.* 1989;9:273-286.

6. Rodger S. A survey of assessments used by paediatric occupational therapists. *Australian Occupational Therapy Journal.* 1994;41:137-142.

7. Polatajko HJ. Results of the Canadian survey. 1998.

8. Burton AW, Miller DE. *Movement skill assessment.* Champaign, IL: Human Kinetics; 1998.

9. Sherrill C. *Adapted Physical Activity, Recreation and Sport: Crossdisciplinary and Lifespan.* 5th ed. Boston: McGraw-Hill; 1998:706.

10. Bruininks RH. *Bruininks-Oseretsky Test of Motor Proficiency: Examiner's Manual.* Circle Pines, MN: American Guidance Service; 1978.

11. Hattie J, Edwards H. A review of the Bruininks-Oseretsky Test of Motor Proficiency. *Br J Educ Psychol.* 1987;57:104-113.

12. Wilson BN, Kaplan BJ, Crawford SG, Dewey D. Interrater Reliability of the Bruininks-Oseretsky Test of Motor Proficiency–Long Form. *Adapt Phys Act Q.* 2000;17:95-110.

13. Henderson SE, Sugden DA. *Movement Assessment Battery for Children.* Kent: The Psychological Corporation; 1992.

14. Stott DH, Moyes FA, Henderson SE. *The Test of Motor Impairment–Henderson Revision.* San Antonio, TX: The Psychological Corporation; 1984.

15. Faraone SF, Biederman J, Milberger S. How reliable are maternal reports of their children's psychopathology? One-year recall of psychiatric diagnoses of ADHD children. *J Am Acad Child Adolesc Psychiatry.* 1995;34:1001.

16. Glascoe FP, Dworkin PH. The role of parents in the detection of developmental and behavioral problems. *Pediatrics.* 1995;95:829-836.

17. Pollock N, Stewart D. Occupational performance needs of school-aged children with physical disabilities in the community. *Physical & Occupational Therapy in Pediatrics.* 1998;18:55-68.

18. Wilson BN, Kaplan BJ, Crawford SC, Campbell A, Dewey D. Reliability and validity of a parent questionnaire on childhood motor skills. *Am J Occup Ther.* in press.

19. Fox MA, Lent B. Clumsy children: Primer on developmental coordination disorder. *Canadian Family Physician.* 1996;42:1965-1971.

20. Miyahara M, Mobs I. Developmental dyspraxia and developmental coordination disorder. *Neuropsychology Review.* 1995;5:245-268.

21. Haley SM, Coster WJ, Ludelow LH, Haltiwanger J, Andrellos PJ. *Pediatric Evaluation of Disability Inventory.* Boston: New England Medical Center Hospitals; 1992.

22. Coster W. Occupation-centered assessment of children. *Am J Occup Ther.* 1998;52:337-344.

23. Riggen KJ, Ulrich DA, Ozmun JC. Reliability and concurrent validity of a test of motor impairment–Henderson revision. *Adapt Phys Act Q.* 1990;7:249-258.

24. Wilson BN. Identification of children and adolescents with Developmental Motor Coordination Disorder. *Telemedicine Canada.* Rehabilitation Therapies; 1998.

25. Dewey D, Wilson BN. Developmental Coordination Disorder: What is it? *Phys Occup Ther Pediatr.* 2001;20:5-27.

26. Wilson BN, Polatajko HJ, Mandich AD, Mcnab JJ. Standardized measures: How well do they indentify children and adolescents with DCD. *World Federation of Occupational Therapy.* Montreal, Canada; 1998.

27. SPSS. *SPSS Base 7.0 Applications Guide.* Chicago: SPSS Inc.; 1996.

28. Kaplan BJ, Wilson BN, Dewey DM, Crawford SG. DCD may not be a discrete disorder. *Human Movement Science.* 1998;17:471-490.

29. Wilson BN, Dewey D, Crawford SG, Kaplan BJ. Reliability and validity of parent questionnaire on childhood motor skills. *Developmental Coordination Disorder: From research to diagnostics and intervention.* 1999:9.

30. Ayres AJ. *Southern California Motor Accuracy Test Manual.* Los Angeles, CA: Western Psychological Services; 1980.

31. Beery KE. *The Developmental Test of Visual-Motor Integration.* 3rd ed. Cleveland: Modern Curriculum Press; 1989.

32. Wechsler D. *Manual for the Wechsler Intelligence Scale for Children–Third Edition.* New York: Psychological Corporation; 1991.

33. Sattler JM. *Assessment of children.* San Diego, CA: Jerome M. Sattler; 1988.

34. Blishen BR, Carroll WK, Moore C. The 1981 socioeconomic index for occupations in Canada. *Can Rev Soc Anthrop.* 1987;24:465-488.

35. Ulrich B. *Test of Gross Motor Development.* Austin, TX: PRO-ED; 1985.

36. Thomas JR, French KE. Gender differences across age in motor performance: A meta-analysis. *Psychol Bull.* 1985;98:260-282.

37. Tirosh E. Fine motor deficit: An etiologically distinct entity. *Pediatr Neurol.* 1994;10:213-216.

38. McConnell D. Processes underlying clumsiness: A review of perspectives. *Phys Occup Ther Pediatr.* 1995;15:33-52.

39. American Psychiatric Association. *Diagnostic and statistical manual of mental disorders.* 4th ed. Washington: American Psychiatric Association; 1994.

40. Broadhead GD, Bruininks RH. Childhood motor performance traits on the short form Bruininks-Oseretsky test. *The Physical Educator.* 1982;39:149-155.

Treatment of Children with Developmental Coordination Disorder: What Is the Evidence?

Angela D. Mandich
Helene J. Polatajko
Jennifer J. Macnab
Linda T. Miller

SUMMARY. Children with Developmental Coordination Disorder (DCD) experience significant difficulty performing everyday tasks and management of these children is a great source of debate. Because little is understood about the etiology of the disorder, treatment design has been driven by competing theories of motor development and motor skill acquisition. Traditional approaches to treatment have been based on neuromaturational, hierarchical theories and, consequently, therapies have focused on remediating underlying deficits with the expecta-

---

Angela D. Mandich, MSc, OT(C), is Instructor, School of Occupational Therapy, and doctoral candidate, School of Kinesiology, The University of Western Ontario, London, Ontario, Canada. Helene J. Polatajko, PhD, OT(C), is Professor and Chair, Department of Occupational Therapy, and Professor, Department of Rehabilitation Science, Faculty of Medicine, University of Toronto, Toronto, Ontario, Canada. Jennifer J. Macnab, BA, PhD Candidate, is affiliated with the Department of Epidemiology & Biostatistics, Faculty of Medicine, The University of Western Ontario, London, Ontario, Canada. Linda T. Miller, PhD, is Assistant Professor, School of Occupational Therapy, Faculty of Health Sciences, The University of Western Ontario, London, Ontario, Canada. All authors are members of the Developmental Coordination Disorder Research Group.

Address correspondence to: Angela D. Mandich, School of Occupational Therapy, The University of Western Ontario, London, Ontario, Canada N6A 5C1.

[Haworth co-indexing entry note]: "Treatment of Children with Developmental Coordination Disorder: What Is the Evidence?" Mandich, Angela D. et al. Co-published simultaneously in *Physical & Occupational Therapy in Pediatrics* (The Haworth Press, Inc.) Vol. 20, No. 2/3, 2001, pp. 51-68; and: *Children with Developmental Coordination Disorder: Strategies for Success* (ed: Cheryl Missiuna) The Haworth Press, Inc., 2001, pp. 51-68. Single or multiple copies of this article are available for a fee from The Haworth Document Delivery Service [1-800-342-9678, 9:00 a.m. - 5:00 p.m. (EST). E-mail address: getinfo@haworthpressinc.com].

tion of subsequent improvement in motor performance. Contemporary approaches, drawn from human movement science, propose that treatment methods be based on the assumption that skill acquisition emerges from the interaction of the child, the task and the environment. This paper provides a review of the treatment literature over the past 15 years, highlighting the fact that little evidence exists to suggest any one approach is better than another. Given current demands for evidence-based practice, and evolving concepts in skill acquisition, a movement toward interventions that are based on functional outcomes is recommended. *[Article copies available for a fee from The Haworth Document Delivery Service: 1-800-342-9678. E-mail address: <getinfo@haworthpressinc.com> Website: <http://www.HaworthPress.com> © 2001 by The Haworth Press, Inc. All rights reserved.]*

KEYWORDS. DCD, intervention, evidence-based practice

INTRODUCTION

I want to ride my bike just like my friends. I want to be able to tie my own shoes. I want my writing to be neat so I can share my favorite journal stories with my friends. I want to hit the baseball, not have the baseball hit me!

Engagement in such typical activities of daily life is an essential component of child development. Indeed, research suggests that participation in childhood activities contributes to the child's cognitive, affective and physical development.[1] However, children with Developmental Coordination Disorder (DCD)[2] have significant functional deficits in activities of daily living and are often referred to therapy to improve performance. In a study of parents' expectations regarding the anticipated outcomes of occupational therapy intervention, Cohn, Miller and Tickle-Degnen[3] found that parents stressed the importance of their children's ability to participate in tasks of daily life. Intervention techniques for children with DCD are varied and the efficacy of these interventions is controversial. Historically, approaches to intervention have focused on remediating underlying processing deficits[4] and facilitating neuromaturational development[5] based upon the assumption that there is a direct relationship between underlying processes and functional performance. More recent theoretical perspectives have questioned this relationship and there has been a resulting increase in interventions that focus directly on skill acquisition and improved performance.

A recent survey of Canadian occupational therapists[6] suggested that therapists often use a combination of these two theoretical perspectives to treat children with DCD. Results of this survey of 116 therapists indicated that the most commonly used therapy approaches included: specific skills training, sensorimotor, functional, compensatory, sensory integration, cognitive behavioral, cognitive, and behavioral (see Figure 1). Not only are a variety of approaches used, but individual therapists use, on average, five different approaches to treat this population of children (see Figure 2).

This survey concurs with the findings of earlier surveys,[7,8] indicating that therapists often use a combination of approaches. Wallen and Walker[7] reported that therapists choose approaches that are based on the child's needs and that given the heterogeneity of DCD, no single approach often works for all children. In the context of increasing emphasis on evidence-based practice,[9,10] therapist preferences provide insufficient rationale for choosing one approach over another. Empirical demonstration of the efficacy of an approach is paramount. The construct of evidence-based practice "de-emphasizes intuition, unsystematic clinical experience, and pathophysiological rationale as

FIGURE 1. Frequency of Use of Different Treatment Approaches (N = 120)

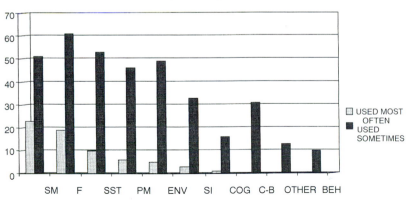

SM = Sensorimotor, F = Functional, SST = Specific Skills Training, PM = Perceptual-Motor, ENV = Environmental, SI = Sensory Integration, COG = Cognitive, C-B = Cognitive Behavioural, B = Behavioural

FIGURE 2. Total Number of Treatment Approaches Used by Clinicians (N = 120)

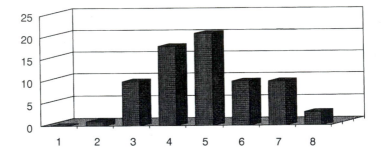

sufficient grounds for clinical decision making and stresses the examination of evidence from clinical research."[9] This shift to evidence-based practice presents many challenges and opportunities for the disciplines of occupational and physical therapy.

An important component of evidence-based practice is the evaluation of the published research on treatment effectiveness. In the case of the treatment of children with DCD, the required evidence for choosing an approach is the effect of the approach on improving motor skill and functional performance. The purpose of this paper is to present a summary of the accumulated evidence for the various treatment approaches to DCD, focusing on the extent to which treatments improve the child's motor performance in daily activities such as bike riding, shoe tying, handwriting, and hitting a baseball.

METHOD

A literature search for intervention and treatment studies was conducted using MEDLINE, PsycINFO, ERIC, and CINAHL, covering the period of 1985-2000. Given that various labels have been used to identify children with DCD,[11, 12] a broad range of key words was used in the search to identify studies of the target population. These keywords included: physically awkward, perceptual-motor dysfunction, developmental coordination disorder, clumsy child syndrome, sensory integration disorder, dyspraxia, apraxia, and motor learning disability.

A total of 46 articles were identified that examined treatment approaches with children with DCD. These included theoretical papers, anecdotal reports of treatment effects, treatment studies, reviews, and surveys. Each treatment study was reviewed and the research design, outcome measures, and results were examined. Considerable variability was found in the rigor of the studies; designs ranged from simple, non-empirical studies to randomized clinical trials; and outcomes ranged from anecdotal descriptions to standardized measures. Although some studies included psychoeducational outcomes as well as measures of motor skill and functional performance, this paper will focus only on treatment studies that reported changes in motor skills and functional outcomes. Thirty-two relevant studies were grouped according to the underlying assumptions of the treatment approach, distinguishing between: (a) "bottom up" approaches that addressed performance components or underlying processes; and, (b) "top down" approaches that focused on skill acquisition and the performance of functional tasks.

RESULTS

Bottom Up Approaches to Intervention

Historically, intervention for children with DCD has been based on neuromaturational theories. These traditional therapies, based on hierarchical theories, have focused on remediating underlying motor deficits with the expectation of subsequent improvement in motor performance.[13] Bottom up approaches that have significantly influenced therapy practice are based on hierarchical theories, which advocate that remediation of underlying deficits results in improved function.[13] With regard to the treatment of children with DCD, bottom up approaches include: (a) sensory integration; (b) process-oriented treatment; (c) perceptual motor training; and (d) combinations of these.

Sensory Integration Intervention

One of the most frequently used approaches to treating DCD is sensory integration (SI).[5] This approach was originally developed for children with a learning disability who had a sensory integrative dysfunction. The SI approach was designed to provide the child with the appropriate sensory stimulation to promote motor adaptation and higher cortical learning. Ayres postulated that sensory input was necessary for optimal function of the brain. Ayres[14] stated "sensory integration is a neurological process that organizes sensation from one's own body and from the environment, and makes it possible to use the body effectively within the environment. The spatial and temporal aspects of inputs from different sensory modalities are interpreted, associated and unified" (p. 11). Ayres maintained that proper sensory input would produce changes in the brain at the neuronal synaptic level. As well, Ayres believed that the nervous system has plasticity and that therapy, primarily in the early childhood years, would promote underlying capabilities and minimize abnormal function. Ayres' original study,[5] a two-group design comparing SI to no treatment, reported that SI therapy improved the academic performance of children with a learning disability. Since this original study, studies comparing the effect of SI therapy to other approaches for a variety of outcomes, including motor and academic performance, have provided little empirical support for SI over other treatments.

Densem, Nutall, Bushnell and Horn[15] studied the effectiveness of SI relative to a physical education program and a no treatment control condition. Children with motor problems were randomly assigned to one of the three groups. No significant difference between groups on measures of language, perceptual motor functioning, reading skills, or handwriting was found as a result of treatment. Similarly, Humphries, Wright, McDougall and Vertes[16] compared three groups, SI therapy, perceptual motor treatment, and no treatment. Thirty children with a learning disability and sensory integrative dysfunction were randomly assigned to one of the three groups. The children in the treatment groups received one hour of intervention per week for 24 weeks. Outcome variables included sensorimotor functioning, cognitive, language, and academic abilities. No significant differences were found in academics, language or cognitive ability. However, the group that received SI therapy made significant gains over the other two groups on measures of sensorimotor functioning.

Polatajko, Law, Miller, Schaffer and Macnab[17] carried out a randomized clinical trial comparing the effectiveness of perceptual motor training and SI in improving the academic and motor performance of children with learning disabilities and sensory integrative dysfunction.

No significance differences were found between groups. Both approaches resulted in improved performance in the motor and academic domains. SI was not found to be superior to perceptual-motor training.

Humphries, Wright, Snider and McDougall[18] compared the effectiveness of SI therapy compared to perceptual motor treatment, and to no treatment with children with learning disability and sensory integrative dysfunction. Children in the treatment groups received 72, one hour sessions, three times per week. Results showed that children who received either SI therapy or perceptual motor treatment improved over the no treatment control group on measures of motor performance. No changes were reported on measures of academic or language ability for either treatment.

Wilson, Kaplan, Fellowes, Gruchy and Faris[19] also investigated the efficacy of SI therapy relative to academic tutoring. No significant differences were found between groups on measures of academics, fine and gross motor skills or visual motor skills. The two treatments were equally effective at improving academic functioning and motor skills. Sensory integration therapy was as effective as tutoring in improving academic functioning and tutoring was as effective as SI in improving motor skills. However, in a follow-up study, Wilson and Kaplan[20] reported that only the SI treatment resulted in sustained gains in gross motor performance for the group that received SI therapy. In an appraisal of these studies, Polatajko, Kaplan and Wilson[21] concluded there is little support for SI as an effective treatment for the academic problems of children with motor and learning disabilities. However, Polatajko, Kaplan and Wilson suggested that with regard to motor skills, SI may be as effective as a perceptual motor approach.

Kaplan, Polatajko, Wilson and Faris[22] examined the efficacy of SI by combining data from two previous studies[17,19] in an effort to increase statistical power. Outcome measures included academic, motor and cognitive abilities. The findings were the same as those for the individual studies; SI therapy, perceptual motor treatment, and tutoring were equally effective in improving academic and motor performance. Hoehn and Baumeister[23] critically appraised the SI literature and questioned the utility and validity of SI for treating children with learning disabilities. They suggested that "the current fund of research findings may well be sufficient to declare SI therapy not merely an unproven but a demonstrably ineffective, primary or adjunctive remedial treatment for learning disabilities and other disorders" (p. 338).

In contrast to the empirical evidence, Stonefelt and Stein[24] reported that parents, teachers and occupational therapists perceived SI therapy to be effective. Using a survey questionnaire, 23 respondents identified SI therapy as extremely or somewhat useful in improving the functional performance of children. Coordination and behavior were the functional areas that were perceived as showing the greatest improvement. However seven of the ten therapists surveyed indicated that they used a combination of several treatment approaches and found these to be more effective than SI alone.

Vargas and Camilli[25] carried out a meta-analysis of SI treatment studies across a number of different populations, including children with a learning disability and sensory integrative dysfunction. Sixteen studies comparing SI with no treatment and 16 studies comparing SI to alternative treatments were included. Results of this meta-analysis were equivocal. When only the earlier studies (1972-1982) were included, SI was found to be more effective than no treatment and equally as effective as various other treatment methods on measures of motor, and psycho-educational ability. However, this effect was not supported in the more recent studies (1983-1993).

In summary, the literature on SI treatment over the last 15 years has focused on comparing the effects of SI to a variety of other approaches including: no treatment, physical education, perceptual motor training, and tutoring. Outcomes have included measures of motor skills, and academic, cognitive, and linguistic performance. The accumulated evidence would suggest that, at best, sensory integration is as effective as any other intervention in improving motor skills. This finding poses a problem for the therapist wishing to present an evidence-based argument for the use of SI over other, less costly, therapies. It also leads to the question of why sensory integration, physical education, perceptual motor training, and tutoring all produce the same effect on motor skills; perhaps these are simply maturational effects. Further, because these studies did not include any functional measures and demonstrated improvements on the motor measures alone, the question of the impact of SI on functional performance remains unanswered. As Humphries et al.[18] noted, gains in motor performance do not seem to generalize to functional skills and abilities.

Process-Oriented Treatment

Another approach used to treat children with motor problems is the process-oriented treatment approach proposed by Laszlo and Bairstow.[4] This approach is based on the premise that kinesthesia is integral to the acquisition and performance of skilled motor behavior.[26,4] Laszlo and Bairstow[4] have suggested that children with DCD have kinesthetic problems and that treatment of these problems will improve motor performance. Their studies,[4,26,27] have reported that process-oriented training can improve motor performance after only eight, 15-minute training sessions.

Hoare and Larkin[28] and Lord and Hulme[29] have questioned the validity of the kinesthetic dysfunction hypothesis, and various others have tried to replicate the findings of Laszlo, Bairstow and colleagues. In a three-group randomized clinical trial of 75 children with DCD, Polatajko et al.[30] compared the process-oriented treatment approach to traditional occupational therapy treatment and no treatment. Results indicated that there was no clear treatment advantage for children in any of the three groups, with only one exception. Children who received the process-oriented approach performed significantly better on the ramp test of the Kinaesthetic Sensitivity Test (KST).

Sims, Henderson, Hulme and Morton[31] compared two groups of 10 clumsy children, one group who received Laszlo and Barstow's process-oriented training and a second group who received no treatment. Improvement in skills as measured by the Test of Motor Impairment and the KST was found in both groups. No significant difference between groups was found. In a subsequent study, Sims, Henderson, Morton and Hulme[32] compared the effect of a cognitive-affective training program with process-oriented training and a no treatment control group. The group that received the process-oriented training showed no advantage relative to the cognitive-affective training group. Sims et al. suggested that general learning principles may be contributing to the observed changes across groups. Based on these findings, Sims and Morton[33] suggest a causal model for skill development that is influenced by cognitive, biological, and motor components.

In summary, the evidence in support of the process-oriented approach is inconclusive. As in the case of SI, some results have indicated that the process-oriented approach is equally as effective as other approaches on measures of kinesthesia and motor skill, whereas others have indicated that it is no better than no treatment at all.

Perceptual-Motor Training

The perceptual-motor approach to the treatment of children with mild motor problems has a long history and continues to be the method of choice for many clinicians.[7] Similar to other bottom up approaches, this approach assumes a causal relationship between motor behavior and underlying perceptual processes. Perceptual-motor training involves providing the child with a broad range of experiences with sensory and motor tasks. General improvement in motor abilities is anticipated as a consequence of enhanced sensory and motor task experience.

Kavale and Mattson[34] conducted a meta-analysis of 180 studies of the effects of perceptual-motor training with children with learning disabilities. Results showed that perceptual-motor training was not effective in remediating the motor difficulties of the children with learning disabilities. Although, there are no recent studies focusing on the perceptual-motor approach, the approach is often included as the contrast group in studies of other approaches, or as part of a combined approach. As previously discussed, all approaches have been found to have comparable effects.

Combined Approaches

A number of the treatment articles that have appeared in the literature describe the use of multiple or combined approaches. In fact therapists (see Figure 2) have reported the use of various combinations of approaches. Although it is not clear how the decision to combine approaches is made, therapists have indicated that they match therapeutic techniques to the individual needs of the child.[7] To date, combined approaches are largely untested. Only two studies addressing combined approaches were found in the last 15 years.

Schoemaker, Hijlkema and Kalverboer[35] evaluated a physiotherapy intervention program that incorporated perceptual-motor training and Bobath techniques.[36] Using a single group design, 18 children participated in a treatment program twice a week, over three months. Improvements were reported in motor skills following the treatment, with benefits maintained at follow up, three months later. Treatment in this study was provided to all children by one therapist.

Rintala, Pienimaki, Ahonen, Cantell, and Kooistra[37] examined the effectiveness of a psychomotor training program for children with a combination of motor and language difficulties. Fifty-four children were divided into two groups and participated in either a 10-week psychomotor training program or a regular physical education program. The Movement Assessment Battery for Children (MABC)[38] and the Test of Gross Motor Development[39] were used as outcome measures. Both groups of children made progress on all measures; however, the psychomotor training group made significantly more gains on object control skills.

In summary, research has provided limited evidence to support combined approaches. Furthermore, Kavale and Mattson[34] noted that, for the most part, combined approaches have demonstrated smaller effects than pure approaches. Taken together, the evidence for bottom up approaches would suggest that no one approach, or combination of approaches, is superior to another in improving motor skill; further, no bottom up approach has been shown to be reliably better than no treatment at all. In summary, the assumed relationship between underlying processes and functional performance has not been confirmed. As Cratty[40] stated, "at this time only the most naive believe in the simple causal relationship between movement capacities, exercise and motor skill and various sensory and perceptual abilities" (p. 201).

Top Down Approaches to Interventions

In contrast to the traditional, neuromaturational theories, recent thinking in movement science has emphasized a problem solving approach to motor skill acquisition.[13] Gentile[13] notes that, "to approach treatment from a movement science framework, the therapist must become an active problem solver utilizing a broad knowledge-base to generate ways of helping a particular patient who is attempting to achieve a specific functional goal" (p. 32). Approaches based on a problem solving premise are only beginning to emerge, and much of the literature in this area is still at a theoretical, non-empirical stage. Recent examples of top down approaches include (a) task specific intervention and (b) cognitive approaches.

Task Specific Intervention

Task specific intervention focuses on direct teaching of the task to be learned. It is based on the premise that performance is the result of learning and that learning is optimal when teaching is focused directly at the target task. Teaching the task is accomplished in steps, including breaking the task down into smaller units, teaching each unit separately, and then linking the units together for whole-task performance. Issues of transfer and generalization are important elements in this approach and must be taught specifically. As Denckla[41] pointed out, "In terms of therapy we have to remember again that many of our motor findings are simply markers and are not directly necessary motor skills that must be remediated. There is no evidence that you get anything other than what you teach. Therapists need to keep in mind the importance of motivation, frustration, fatigue and boredom" (p. 254).

In an early descriptive study of task specific intervention, Hawkins and Gadsby[42] treated individuals with motor problems, focusing on teaching concepts and basic skills, fostering generalization, and building confidence. Although this study was limited by a small sample size and the lack of standardized measures, Hawkins and Gadsby reported improvements in self-confidence and skills. Using a two-group experimental design, Revie and Larkin[43] investigated the use of task specific intervention for treating children with motor problems. Twenty-four children were taught either to throw a ball and hop, or to catch and bounce a volleyball and target kick. Children received one-hour sessions, twice a week for four weeks. Task specific training resulted in significant gains for each group although transfer to other tasks was not observed. This finding of a task specific intervention effect, without transfer, is consistent with the observation described earlier of Polatajko et al.[30] that the only significant effect of the process-oriented approach was the ramp task of the KST, where task specific training was apparent.

Cognitive Approaches

In recent years, a number of different cognitive approaches have been proposed. Bouffard and Wall[6] proposed a problem-solving framework to guide skill acquisition. Bouffard and Wall[44] postulate that five inter-related steps guide motor skill acquisition. In the initial step, Problem Identification, the child identifies the nature of the problem to be solved. In the next step, Problem Representation, the child generates an appropriate, accurate, depiction of the motor problem. This precise representation is necessary for the child to plan and reach the final goal. Third, in Plan Construction, the child forms a plan to solve the movement problem and explores alternatives. Plan construction is described as a complex process that may require evaluation and revision of the plan until a suitable plan emerges. In the fourth step, Plan Execution, the child executes the plan. At this stage, success may be achieved if an appropriate plan was chosen and executed. Evaluation of Progress, the final step, occurs during and after the plan has been performed. Bouffard and Wall's problem solving approach has not been empirically tested to date.

Henderson and Sugden[38] proposed a similar approach to that of Bouffard and his colleagues.[44] Henderson and Sugden's model, the Cognitive Motor Approach, is based on an information-processing framework and consists of a three-step process of motor skill acquisition. The initial step, Movement Planning, requires the child to evaluate whether or not the task is attainable. In order to do this, the child must understand the task and its demands. The child acquires this information through sensory and perceptual processes, including vision and kinesthesia, then transforms this information into a plan. After establishing a clear expectation of the task demands the child proceeds to the second step, Movement Execution. The child uses the plan to guide execution of the movement. This step involves several factors, including spatial considerations, force and sequencing, and organization of movement. During the final step, Movement Evaluation, the child monitors his/her progress. Using the cognitive motor approach, Wright and Sugden[45] demonstrated that this intervention was beneficial in improving the functional skills of children with DCD. Using a one-group design, 18 children with DCD participated in a five-week intervention program that was tailored to each child's individual needs. Using the Movement Assessment Battery for Children as an outcome measure, significant improvements from pretest to posttest were found.

A third cognitive approach, the Cognitive Orientation to daily Occupational Performance, (CO-OP) has been proposed by Polatajko and colleagues.[46] This approach has it roots in Meichenbaum's[47] problem solving, verbal self-instructional program. CO-OP is a child-centred approach that focuses on increasing functional performance through strategy use. In this approach, generalization and transfer of skills is promoted through the ecological relevance of the tasks being addressed, the mediational techniques that are used and parent involvement. This issue contains a description of CO-OP,[46] and a summary of the research to date.[46] As detailed in the articles in this issue and in Miller, Polatajko, Missiuna, Mandich, MacNab,[48] the evidence suggests that CO-OP is an effective approach to increase the functional performance of children with DCD. However, it should be noted that CO-OP has only been accessible through the literature for a brief period of time and as yet, there has been no independent evaluation of the approach.

Although top-down approaches are congruent with contemporary motor learning theories and appear promising, the evidence regarding their potential to improve the motor skills and functional performance of children with DCD is only beginning to accumulate.

DISCUSSION

Children with DCD experience significant difficulty in performing everyday tasks, which often results in a referral to therapy. In Cohn, Miller and Tickle-Degnen's[3] survey of expectations for outcomes of occupational therapy, parents emphasized their desire to see changes in the functional performance of their children as an outcome of treatment. Parents' expectations are consistent with Coster's[49] and Trombly's[50] advocacy for a top-down approach to intervention, beginning with the occupations that the person needs to perform.

Intervention for children with DCD has been a great source of debate. Because little is understood about the etiology of the disorder, treatment design has been driven by competing theories of motor development and motor skill acquisition. Gentile[13] noted "the assumptions underlying therapeutic approaches based on movement science are not reconciled with those underlying traditional, neurotherapies based on a facilitation model" (p. 32).

Current theories of skill acquisition emphasize the importance of contextual factors over neuromaturational factors in motor skill acquisition. Gentile[13] suggested that skill acquisition is a function of the interaction between the environment, the child and task and argued that if the goal is to facilitate skill acquisition in children, it may be fruitful to pursue interventions based on functional activities, rather than of focusing on underlying components. Other authors[51,52,53] also support this task-oriented approach. It would appear from this review that the evidence required to settle this controversy is not yet available.

Although bottom up approaches have a long tradition, the empirical data do not convincingly support their effectiveness in improving the motor skills of children with DCD, nor do they support the assumed relationship between underlying processes and functional performance. Many of the studies reporting support for this approach have methodological weakness and are often limited by small sample size, lack of a control group or randomization, and use of measures lacking in reliability and validity. Where well-controlled studies do exist, they tend not to support this approach.

The top down approaches, on the other hand, are relatively new and studies of their effectiveness are only beginning to appear. Early evidence for the use of top down approaches with a DCD population, and collateral evidence from other populations, suggests that these approaches may be very effective in teaching specific tasks and in improving the functional performance of children with DCD. An important question to be addressed will be that of generalization and skill transfer; as well, larger studies are needed.

In the absence of strong evidence, therapists must rely on their clinical judgment to determine the best approach. Therapists do this by individualizing therapy, often combining a number of approaches, depending on the needs of the particular child being treated. Although this seems to make good clinical sense, on a case-by-case basis, it precludes the accumulation of sufficient evidence to argue for the efficacy of a treatment approach and this makes it difficult to launch an evidence-based argument for best practice. It will be important for us to develop a systematic, evidence-based approach to the treatment of these children.

Fisher[54] discussed meaningful occupation as a powerful therapeutic agent and suggested that measuring functional/occupational outcomes is imperative. Combining the idea of measuring functional outcomes with current theories of motor learning may provide therapists with insights into the understanding and management of the problems experienced by children with DCD.

REFERENCES

1. Manning ML. Play development from ages eight to twelve. In: Fromberg DP, Bergen D. eds. *Play from birth to twelve and beyond: contexts, perspectives, and meanings.* New York, NY: Garland; 1998.

2. American Psychiatric Association. Motor skills disorder 315.40. Developmental coordination disorder. *Diagnostic and statistical manual of mental disorders (DSM-IV).* 4th ed. Washington, DC: Author 1994:53-55.

3. Cohn E, Miller LJ, Tickle-Degnen L. Parental hopes for therapy outcomes: children with sensory modulation disorders. *Am J Occup Ther* 2000;54(1):36-43.

4. Laszlo JI, Bairstow PJ. *Perceptual-motor behaviour: developmental assessment and therapy.* New York, NY: Praeger; 1985.

5. Ayres AJ. *Sensory integration and learning disorders.* Los Angeles, CA: Western Psychological Services; 1972.

6. Mandich A, Polatajko HJ, Miller L, Macnab J, Missiuna C. Cognitive strategies–getting DCD kids to succeed: from research to diagnostics and intervention. *Fourth biannual workshop on children with developmental coordination disorder programme.* Groenigen, Holland; October 7-8th, 1999.

7. Wallen M, Walker R. Occupational therapy practice with children with perceptual motor dysfunction: findings of a literature review and survey. *Australian Occup Ther J* 1995;42:15-25.

8. Yack E. Sensory integration: a survey of its use in the clinical setting. *Can J Occup Ther* 1989;56(5):229-235.

9. Evidence-Based Medicine Working Group. Evidence-based medicine: a new approach to teaching the practice of medicine. *J Am Med Assoc* 1992;268(17): 2420-2425.

10. Law M, Baum C. Evidence-based occupational therapy practice. *Can J Occup Ther* 1998; 65:131-135.

11. Missiuna C, Polatajko HJ. Developmental dyspraxia by any other name: are they all just clumsy? *Am J Occup Ther* 1995; 49:619-627.

12. Polatajko HJ. Developmental coordination disorder (DCD) alias the clumsy child. In: *A neurodevelopmental approach to specific learning disorders.* London, UK: MacKeith 1997:119-133

13. Gentile AM. The nature of skill acquisition: therapeutic implications for children with movement disorders. *Med Sport Sci* 1992; 36:31-40.

14. Ayres AJ. *Sensory integration and praxis tests.* Los Angeles, CA: Western Psychological Services; 1989.

15. Densem JF, Nuthall A, Bushnell J, Horn J. Effectiveness of a sensory integrative program for children with perceptual-motor deficits. *J Learning Disabil* 1989; 22(4):221-229.

16. Humphries TW, Wright M, McDougall B, Vertes J. The efficacy of sensory integration therapy for children with learning disability. *Phys & Occup Ther Peds* 1990;10(3):1-17.

17. Polatajko HJ, Law M, Miller J, Schaffer R, Macnab JJ. The effect of a sensory integration program on academic achievement, motor performance, and self-esteem in children identified as learning disabled: results of a clinical trial. *Occup Ther J Res* 1991;11:155-176.

18. Humphries TW, Wright M, Snider L, McDougall B. A comparison of the effectiveness of sensory integration therapy and perceptual motor training in treating children with learning disabilities. *J Dev Behavior Peds* 1992; 13:31-40.

19. Wilson BN, Kaplan BJ, Fellowes S, Gruchy C, Faris P. The efficacy of sensory integration treatment compared to tutoring. *Phys & Occup Ther Peds* 1992;12(1): 1-35.

20. Wilson BN, Kaplan BJ. Follow-up assessment of children receiving sensory integration treatment. *Occup Ther J Res* 1994; 14(4):244-266.

21. Polatajko HJ, Kaplan BJ, Wilson B. Sensory integration treatment for children with learning disabilities: its status 20 years later. *Occup Ther J Res* 1992;12(6): 323-339.

22. Kaplan BJ, Polatajko HJ, Wilson BN, Faris PD. Reexamination of sensory integration treatment: a combination of two efficacy studies. *J Learning Disabil* 1993; 26(5):342-347.

23. Hoehn TP, Baumeister AA. A critique of the application of sensory integration therapy to children with learning disabilities. *J Learning Disabilities* 1994;27(6): 338-350.

24. Stonefelt LL, Stein F. Sensory integrative techniques applied to children with learning disabilities: an outcome study. *Occup Ther Internat* 1998;5(4):252-272.

25. Vargas S, Camilli G. A meta-analysis of research on sensory integration treatment. *Am J Occup Ther* 1999; 53(2):189-198.

26. Bairstow PJ, Laszlo JI. Deficits in the planning, control and recall of hand movements in children with perceptuo-motor dysfunction. *British J Dev Psychol* 1989;7:251-253

27. Laszlo JI, Bairstow PJ, Bartrip J, Rolfe UT. Clumsiness or perceptuo-motor dysfunction? In: Colley AM, Beech JR. eds. *Cognition and action in skilled behaviour.* North-Holland: Elsevier Science BV; 1988.

28. Hoare D, Larkin D. Kinaesthetic abilities of clumsy children. *Dev Med Child Neurol* 1991; 33: 671-678.

29. Lord R, Hulme C. Perceptual judgment of normal and clumsy children. *Dev Med Child Neurol* 1987; 29:250-257.

30. Polatajko H.J, Macnab JJ, Anstett B, Malloy-Miller T, Murphy K, Noh S. A clinical trial of the process-oriented treatment approach for children with developmental co-ordination disorder. *Dev Med Child Neurol* 1995; 37:310-319.

31. Sims K, Henderson SE, Hulme C, Morton J. The remediation of clumsiness: an evaluation of Laszlo's kinaesthetic approach [part one]. *Dev Med Child Neurol* 1996; 38(11):976-987.

32. Sims K, Henderson SE, Morton J, Hulme C. The remediation of clumsiness: is kinaesthesis the answer? [part two]. *Dev Med Child Neurol* 1996;38(11):988-997.

33. Sims K, Morton J. Modelling the training effects of kinaesthetic acuity measurement. *J Child Psychol Psych* 1998;39(5):731-746.

34. Kavale K, Mattson D. "One jumped off the balance beam": meta-analysis of perceptual-motor training. *J Learning Disabil* 1983; 16(3):165-173.

35. Schoemaker MM, Hijlkema MGJ, Kalverboer AF. Physiotherapy for clumsy children: an evaluation study. *Dev Med Child Neurol* 1994; 36:143-155.

36. Bobath K, Bobath B. The neuro-developmental treatment. In: Scrutton, D. ed. *Management of Motor Disorders of Children with Cerebral Palsy, Clinics in Developmental Medicine*, No. 90. London: S.I.M.P; 1984.

37. Rintala P, Pienimaki K, Ahonen T, Cantell M, Kooistra L. The effects of a psychomotor training programme on motor skill development in children with developmental language disorders. *Human Movement Sci* 1998; 17:721-737.

38. Henderson SE, Sugden D. *The Movement Assessment Battery for Children.* Kent, UK: Psychological Corp.; 1992.

39. Ulrich DA. *Test of gross motor development.* Austin, TX: Pro-Ed; 1985.

40. Cratty BJ. *Clumsy child syndromes description, evaluation and remediation.* USA: Harwood Academic; 1994.

41. Denckla MB. Developmental dyspraxia: the clumsy child. In: Levine MD, Satz P. eds. *Middle childhood: development and dysfunction.* Baltimore, MD: University Park Press; 1984.

42. Hawkins S, Gadsby M. Perceptual-motor deficit: a major learning difficulty. *British J Occup Ther* 1991; 54(4):145-149.

43. Revie G, Larkin D. Task-specific intervention with children reduces movement problems. *Adapt Phys Activ Quar* 1993; 10:29-41.

44. Bouffard M, Wall AE. A problem solving approach to movement skill acquisition: implications for special populations. In: Reid G. ed. *Problems in movement control.* North-Holland: Elsevier Science; 1990.

45. Wright HC, Sugden DA. A school based intervention programme for children with developmental coordination disorder. *European J Physical Educ* 1998;3:35-50.

46. Polatajko HJ, Mandich AD, Miller LT, Macnab JJ.Cognitive orientation to daily occupational performance (CO-OP): Part II–The evidence. *Phys Occup Ther Peds* 2001;20(2/3):83-106.

47. Meichenbaum D. *Cognitive-behavior modification: an integrative approach.* New York, NY: Plenum; 1997.

48. Miller L, Polatajko HJ, Missiuna C, Mandich A, Macnab JJ. A pilot trial of a cognitive treatment for children with developmental coordination disorder. *Human Movement Science* [accepted].

49. Coster W. Occupation-centered assessment of children. *Am J Occup Ther* 1998;52(5):337-344.

50. Trombly C. Anticipating the future: assessment of occupational function. *Am J Occup Ther* 1993;47(3):253-257.

51. Mathiowetz V, Haugen JB. Motor behavior research: implications for therapeutic approaches to central nervous system dysfunction. *Am J Occup Ther* 1994; 48(8):733-744.

52. Thelen E. Self-organization in developmental process: can systems approaches work? In: Gunner M, Thelen E. eds. *The Minnesota symposium in child psychology.* Hillsdale, NJ: Lawrence Erlbaum; 1998.

53. Ulrich BD. Dynamic systems theory and skill development in infants and children. In: Connolly KJ, Forssberg H. eds. *Neurophysiology and Neuropsychology of Motor Development.* London, UK: Cambridge University Press; 1997.

54. Fisher AG. Uniting practice and theory: an occupational therapy framework [1998 Eleanor Clarke Slagle Lecture]. *Am J Occup Ther* 1998; 52:509-521.

Cognitive Orientation to Daily Occupational Performance (CO-OP): Part I– Theoretical Foundations

Cheryl Missiuna
Angela D. Mandich
Helene J. Polatajko
Theresa Malloy-Miller

SUMMARY. This paper is the first in a series of three papers that present the systematic development and evaluation of Cognitive Orien-

Cheryl Missiuna, PhD, OT(C), is Assistant Professor, School of Rehabilitation Science, and Co-Investigator, CanChild Centre for Childhood Disability Research, McMaster University, Hamilton, Ontario, Canada. Angela D. Mandich, MSc, OT(C), is a doctoral candidate, School of Kinesiology, and Instructor, School of Occupational Therapy, The University of Western Ontario, London, Ontario, Canada. Helene J. Polatajko, PhD, OT(C), is Professor and Chair, Department of Occupational Therapy, and Professor, Faculty of Education, The University of Western Ontario, London, Ontario, Canada. Theresa Malloy-Miller, MSc, OT(C), is Occupational Therapist, Thames Valley Children's Centre, London, Ontario, Canada. All authors are members of the Developmental Coordination Disorder Research Group.

Address correspondence to: Cheryl Missiuna, PhD, OT(C), School of Rehabilitation Science, Institute of Applied Health Sciences, McMaster University, 1400 Main Street West, Hamilton, Ontario, Canada L8S 1C7 (E-mail: missiuna@mcmaster.ca).

The authors gratefully acknowledge the support of the Edith Herman Research Fund in the preparation of this manuscript.

Selected portions of this manuscript are similar in content to an article written by the authors that was published in the *Canadian Journal of Occupational Therapy*, Volume 65(4), and are reproduced with permission.

[Haworth co-indexing entry note]: "Cognitive Orientation to Daily Occupational Performance (CO-OP): Part I–Theoretical Foundations." Missiuna, Cheryl et al. Co-published simultaneously in *Physical & Occupational Therapy in Pediatrics* (The Haworth Press, Inc.) Vol. 20, No. 2/3, 2001, pp. 69-81; and: *Children with Developmental Coordination Disorder: Strategies for Success* (ed: Cheryl Missiuna) The Haworth Press, Inc., 2001, pp. 69-81. Single or multiple copies of this article are available for a fee from The Haworth Document Delivery Service [1-800-342-9678, 9:00 a.m. - 5:00 p.m. (EST). E-mail address: getinfo@haworthpressinc.com].

tation to daily Occupational Performance (CO-OP). CO-OP is a cognitively based, child-centred intervention that enables children to achieve their functional goals. In Part I, the breadth of literature that provides the theoretical underpinnings for the approach is reviewed. Parts II and III provide a description of the approach and present the evidence to support its use with children with developmental coordination disorder. *[Article copies available for a fee from The Haworth Document Delivery Service: 1-800-342-9678. E-mail address: <getinfo@haworthpressinc.com> Website: <http://www.HaworthPress.com> © 2001 by The Haworth Press, Inc. All rights reserved.]*

KEYWORDS. DCD, rehabilitation, therapy, functional outcomes

Nearly a decade ago, when it became apparent that the intervention approaches which had been used in pediatric therapy were relatively ineffective with children with developmental coordination disorder (DCD), a number of researchers determined that it was time to develop a new frame of reference, a new way of approaching intervention with these children.[1,2] In the early 1990s, Polatajko and colleagues (see parts II and III in this volume) set out to develop a new approach to the treatment of children with DCD. Ideally, therapeutic interventions are based upon our knowledge of the population of children to be served, are grounded in associated theories of disability and treatment, and are systematically tested, refined and elucidated. A series of questions, therefore, needed to be addressed.

First, what did we know about children with DCD? Research studies conducted with these children had produced some very interesting observations. Children with DCD were consistently delayed in the acquisition of motor skills, but their intellectual abilities did not seem to be affected.[3,4] Although they were able to learn both novel and familiar motor tasks, they never reached the level of proficiency of their age-matched, non-DCD peers.[5] Further, for some unexplainable reason, children with DCD appeared to continue to perform a task the same way, over and over again, whether it was successful or not.[6,7] They seemed to have difficulty selecting a motor response that would be appropriate for any given situation[8,9] and, even when they had learned a skill, seemed to be unable to transfer or generalize it to other tasks or environments.[5,10] All of these observations appeared to be consistent with the idea that children with DCD have difficulty learning and generalizing motor skills. If one assumes that motor skills need to be learned and retained in a similar fashion to other types of skills, then it seems reasonable to explore this as a problem of skill acquisition.

Secondly, we asked what theories of treatment might be appropriate, given the nature of the disability? In order to develop a cohesive approach that would guide intervention with these children, theories were sought that might provide a foundation for a new acquisition-based approach. The theories that provide guidance for a cognitive, or problem-solving, orientation arise from the fields of cognitive and educational psychology. In recent years, it has become evident that these theories are also entirely compatible with the evolution of theory that has taken place in the fields of motor learning and motor control. When this theoretical frame of reference is applied within occupational therapy, then additional thought needs to be given to models of client-centred practice. Finally, since cognitive strategies are an important aspect of problem-solving interventions, theories regarding the teaching and use of strategies also need to be considered. The purpose of this paper is to provide a concise overview of the theories that have served to provide the foundation for the cognitive approach to intervention, the Cognitive Orientation to daily Occupational Performance (CO-OP), that is described in parts two and three of this series.

THEORIES OF LEARNING AND PROBLEM-SOLVING*

Many theories within cognitive and educational psychology can be traced back to the writings of L. S. Vygotsky (1896-1934). Vygotsky[11] was a Russian psychologist who spent time observing the problem-solving attempts of young children. He noted that, during problem-solving tasks (e.g., when children were asked to draw but not given crayons), young children spoke aloud at points of difficulty. In contrast, older children appeared to think about a solution, then act. When children were asked about their problem-solving, however, it became apparent that the thoughts of the older children were very similar to

---

*The theories within this section only were previously reviewed by the authors in the publication, Missiuna C, Malloy-Miller T, Mandich A. Mediational techniques: Origins and application to occupational therapy in pediatrics. *Cdn Jour Occup Ther.* 1998; 65(4), 202-209. A summarized version of that review is reproduced here with permission.

the overt speech used by the younger children. Vygotsky[11] concluded that children need to be able to talk themselves through a problem and that this served to help the child formulate a plan. Vygotsky believed that cognitive development occurred through the gradual internalization of concepts and relationships that were learned through interaction with others who were more cognitively competent. He suggested that children first experience cognitive activities such as problem-solving in situations in which there is a child, an activity, and a significant other. The adult initially does most of the cognitive work; however, gradually the adult's speech is internalized by the child and, with experience and application, becomes part of the child's repertoire.

Luria,[12,13] a student of Vygotsky, further detailed the process involved when one is learning a new concept or exploring a problem. He suggested that there were five stages to the problem-solving process: (1) discovery of the problem; (2) investigation of the problem; (3) selection of alternative solutions; (4) attempt to solve the problem; (5) comparison of results of the solution. Luria[12,13] strongly supported Vygotsky's belief that a child initially talks aloud to direct problem-solving and that the steps of the process are then rehearsed by the child internally as covert speech. It was this aspect of Vygotsky's work–the use of internal speech to guide and regulate one's behaviour–that Meichenbaum drew upon to develop his ideas for cognitive-behavioural approaches.

Meichenbaum[14,15] proposed that a child could learn to regulate his behaviour by instructing himself to identify a goal, develop a plan, enact the plan, and evaluate its success. Meichenbaum and Goodman[16] described a series of self-instructional steps in which problem-solving stages would be modeled by a competent adult, then stated aloud by the child, then internalized and recalled covertly by the child. Meichenbaum[15] outlined a problem-solving structure that could be easily learned by the child because it had just four simple steps, Goal-Plan-Do-Check, that were similar to the stages described earlier by Luria.[13] In order to ensure that this problem-solving structure would be learned and generalized by the child, Meichenbaum emphasized the importance of scaffolding the child's learning, i.e., using everyday activities, learning the structure in a context in which it could be used, bridging to other real life examples, individualizing the plan and having a significant adult provide feedback to the child.

While this type of global problem-solving structure was being detailed in North America, Feuerstein and colleagues in Israel were delineating the type of adult guidance that would be needed to foster cognitive development and problem-solving within a child.[17] Feuerstein believed that cognitive development resulted from two types of interactions: the first, direct exposure to tasks within the environment, was consistent with Piagetian models of development. The second type of interaction that Feuerstein believed to be essential was a newer idea that was termed "mediated learning experience."[17,18] He believed that daily experiences needed to be interpreted by an adult who would select and organize environmental stimuli until it was appropriate for the child's level of learning. Feuerstein assumed that any "deficiency" in the child or the environment that appeared to hinder learning (e.g., motor or learning problems, poverty) was only of secondary concern since that deficiency might not be able to be changed. He suggested that the essential factor determining whether or not a child's cognitive abilities could be improved was the presence of a mediator, someone who would be able to help the child make sense out of his or her life experiences.[19] Becoming a mediator meant that the adult would take an active role as an intermediary between the child and the task, assisting the child to derive a more generalized meaning from it. Feuerstein et al.[19] and subsequently Haywood[20,21] outlined the techniques that would be used by an adult in order to mediate effectively with a child. These interactive techniques include process questioning, bridging, comparison/describing, modeling, challenging and elaborated feedback (for a detailed description, please see Missiuna, Malloy-Miller, and Mandich[22]).

In Cognitive Orientation to daily Occupational Performance (CO-OP, described in detail in Polatajko et al., this volume), Vygotsky's belief that a child needs to guide him or herself through problem-solving by talking aloud is strongly maintained. Meichenbaum's problem solving structure–Goal, Plan, Do, Check–is used as the global strategy that is applied to every daily task that the child works on in therapy and many of his ideas about how to teach this approach to children have been retained. These ideas are combined with the mediational techniques outlined by Feuerstein and Haywood to facilitate guided discovery and provide the method through which the therapist elicits responses from the child and bridges that learning to other daily living situations.

THEORIES OF MOTOR LEARNING AND MOTOR CONTROL

Since the 1960s, motor learning and motor control theories have been grounded in the idea that changes in motor behaviour and skill occurred as a result of maturation of the central nervous system. This system was originally believed to be organized hierarchically with the cortex gradually gaining control over primitive reflexes and integrating these to produce functional movement patterns.[23] Back in 1967, Bernstein[24] had proposed that motor learning should be thought of as a process of solving movement problems. Practice of a motor skill, according to Bernstein, was not meant to be for the purpose of repeating the solution to a motor problem but in order to repeat, and learn, the process needed to solve it. For the next twenty years, Bernstein's ideas were largely overlooked as theorists continued to support hierarchical models of motor learning. Schmidt,[25] for example, proposed that generalized motor programs resided within the central nervous system that stored the initial conditions of a movement, the parameters that were used to make it and the results of the movement. New movement patterns were generated during practice of the movement as feedback was utilized to specify and refine parameters such as force and distance. Schmidt's theories reinforced the hierarchical view of motor learning; however, they also contributed significantly to our understanding of the importance of knowing and learning from the outcome of a movement, called "knowledge of results."[26]

In the 1990s, we have seen a strong return to the type of thinking originally espoused by Bernstein.[24] Modern day theorists argue against the idea that motor patterns are formed and represented hierarchically. Instead, they suggest that motor control and development emerge as a result of the interaction of multiple, cooperative systems as the child tries to solve movement problems.[27] These theories, captured by the term "dynamic systems theories," propose that the systems of the person–musculoskeletal, neural, cognitive–interact with the person's motivation to perform the task, with the structure and requirements of the task itself and within the constraints of the environment.[28] New movements and motor control result from the collaboration of all of these parts of the system as they organize themselves in order to solve a movement problem. The parameters of the task, the environment, and the level of readiness of the child influence the type of learning that can take place and the movement strategies that will be developed.[29] If a therapist wants to facilitate motor learning, he or she has to determine the factors that might be changed in order to move the system forward.[30] In some instances, these factors may involve trying to change the positioning or body mechanics of the child. In other instances, however, factors such as practice, knowledge about the task and motivation to improve performance may have more impact.[31]

Gentile[32] recently described two types of learning processes that she believes occur concurrently during the acquisition of a functional motor skill. Explicit learning processes take place as the child consciously attempts to put into place a known movement that will approximate the demands of the task. For example, if a child has already learned how to catch a beach ball, he will have a general idea of the body and arm position that might be required to catch a basketball. With practice, postural stability, specific joint positioning, muscle contraction patterns and other forces become more refined through a process called implicit learning. Explicit learning, since it is a conscious process, may be able to be facilitated through verbal instruction whereas it is probable that implicit learning is less accessible to this type of intervention.[32]

In CO-OP, the child is learning a new motor skill or improving performance on one that has not yet developed sufficiently to be functional for the child. If motor learning is viewed as the child solving a movement problem[29] then children need to learn the process involved in discovering a solution for themselves.[33] This type of problem-solving involves generating alternative ways of solving the movement problem and then "discovering" which method works most efficiently. Guided discovery is described in more detail in the next section and in subsequent papers. It involves the therapist setting up the environment to draw the child's attention to the specific point at which he or she is getting stuck, to discover the relevant features of the task, the environment and their body and then to generate alternative solutions to the movement(s) that the child is currently using. In this way, appropriate movement strategies will become evident to the child.

CHILD-CENTRED INTERVENTION AND CHILD-CHOSEN GOALS

The interaction of the individual, the task and the environment that has been emphasized recently in motor learning theories has been stressed with equal importance in occupational therapy literature. Numerous theorists have identified that successful performance of daily activities results from an optimal match between the person, the environment and the occupation (e.g.,[34,35,36,37]). While this may seem to be an obvious observation, this way of thinking about maximizing performance has moved us toward prioritizing intervention that focuses on the goal or task itself, rather than on the component skills and abilities that are believed to underlie performance of the task. Traditionally, therapists might have analysed the tasks or goals that were selected by the child, identified underlying component deficits (e.g., eye hand coordination difficulties, poor balance) and then remediated those areas. This "bottom-up" approach[38] was grounded in the hierarchical models of neurodevelopment, referred to earlier, that suggested that motor control would emerge when underlying skills were adequately developed.[39] With the advent of dynamic systems theories of motor learning, therapists such as Mathiewitz and Haugen[40] have suggested that, because motor learning is a multistage process of interaction between the individual, the environment, and the occupation, motor control will emerge as the individual becomes more efficient and effective at performing a specific task.[40] Intervention approaches that begin and end with an emphasis upon the child's selected goal have therefore been referred to as "top-down"[38] or "occupation based" approaches.[41]

Focusing on child-chosen goals is also important from the perspective of the ecological relevance of the task. Bandura[42,43,44] has suggested that children's actual experiences performing an activity contribute most significantly to their self-perceptions. As children develop metacognitive abilities, they become able to reflect upon their task performance and to judge their capabilities and limitations quite accurately. When children identify areas of difficulty and then set goals, they usually feel empowered.[43,45] These feelings of empowerment lead to increased goal commitment which may, in turn, increase performance and perceived competence and foster the setting of new goals.[46] Children also become able to consider how expenditure of effort, persistence and other factors can compensate for lack of ability.[44]

In CO-OP, a child-centred approach is taken and children are encouraged to select their own goals for intervention. At the age at which children participate in CO-OP, their metacognitive skills are developed sufficiently for them to be able to consider their task performance across situations. They are motivated to work on achieving goals that they have set personally.

THEORIES OF STRATEGY USE

A related body of literature that provides underpinnings for this approach is drawn from the work of Pressley and colleagues[47,48,49] on the use of cognitive strategies to facilitate learning. Strategies have been defined as "an individual's approach to a task when it includes how a person thinks and acts when planning, executing and evaluating performance on a task and its outcomes" (p. 5).[50] This planful approach to task performance is potentially conscious and may involve the implementation of both cognitive and metacognitive strategies. Normally, cognitive strategies are put in place efficiently and automatically in order to plan and execute a task. When the task becomes difficult, relative to the child's skill level, then metacognitive (or executive) strategies are required to select appropriate cognitive strategies, monitor and evaluate their application. Implementing these metacognitive strategies involves going through the problem solving structure described earlier. Once strategy use becomes automatic and efficient, then metacognition, thinking about and monitoring the strategies consciously, will no longer be necessary.[49] Like Meichenbaum, Borkowski and colleagues have argued in favour of the child using self-instructional routines to guide their problem solving as these routines "force the child to consider the demands of both the task and the strategy and to match the strategy to the task on the basis of shared features"(p. 66).[49]

Concepts implicit in strategy instruction address the question of transfer and generalization very directly. In order to generalize a strategy, the child must have knowledge of how, when and where to use the strategy.[48] The optimal way to facilitate transfer is inherent in the method of learning the strategies in the first place. Pressley and colleagues recommend guided discovery learning which involves posing questions to the child that focus on factors that are relevant and irrelevant in order to help children figure out the relevant cues. They then ask the child to form and state a cognitive rule that includes specifying the conditions that must be in place for that strategy to apply. Guided discovery is remarkably similar to the scaffolding concepts of Meichenbaum and the mediational techniques described by Feuerstein and Haywood who recommend the use of process questions–questions that focus on the problem solving process and that highlight relevant features of the task. All groups of theorists emphasize the importance of individual instruction being provided at the level of the child's skill. Application of a strategy across tasks facilitates transfer but generalization to other learning situations must be addressed as well. Pressley and colleagues believe that guided discovery facilitates transfer and generalization because the child obtains a more complete understanding of the strategies and their usage. Feuerstein et al. have suggested the importance of the mediator "bridging," deliberately asking questions that prompt the child to think about other times when that task might be performed or that strategy might be useful.

In CO-OP, cognitive strategies are used to influence skill acquisition. Generalization and transfer of skills is supported through the use of an executive, or problem-solving strategy, that trains the child to monitor his performance and self-evaluate the outcome. Domain-specific strategies form the bridge between the child's ability and skill level and help them to develop appropriate motor plans.

CONCLUSIONS

Kramer and Hinojosa[51] indicate that the theoretical base "sets the stage for the entire frame of reference" (p. 73) of an approach to intervention and outlines the relationship between all of its elements. The elements of CO-OP include theories regarding problem-solving, children's learning, motor learning, cognitive strategies, client-centred practice, goal setting and motivation: they are drawn from many different fields but are internally consistent with one another in providing a foundation for a cognitive approach to intervention. The literature reviewed in this paper provides support for the following conclusions:

a. Current motor learning theories offer support for an approach that focuses on child-chosen goals. Motor control can be expected to emerge as a child works on a task that he or she is motivated to learn;

b. Goals, or tasks, will need to be ecologically valid, performed in a realistic setting, with practice opportunities and feedback focusing on the child learning to solve movement problems;

c. A global problem-solving structure will be needed that will develop the child's ability to select, apply, evaluate and monitor task-specific cognitive strategies;

d. In order to facilitate transfer and generalization of learned strategies, the child will need to be guided to discover these strategies and encouraged, through questioning, to focus on the process of selecting them and on evaluating their outcome.

The next step in developing a model for practice is described in Part II of this series and involves the systematic development and testing of a protocol for intervention with children with DCD.

REFERENCES

1. Bouffard M, Wall AE. A problem solving approach to movement skill acquisition: Implications for special populations. In: Reid G, ed. *Problems in movement control.* North-Holland: Elsevier Science; 1990.

2. Henderson SE, Sugden D. *The Movement Assessment Battery for Children.* London: Psychological Corp; 1992.

3. Wall AE, Reid G, Paton, J. The syndrome of physical awkwardness. In: Reid G, ed. *Problems in movement control.* North-Holland: Elsevier Science; 1990.

4. Polatajko HJ. Developmental Coordination Disorder (DCD) alias the clumsy child. In: Willems GW, ed. *A Neurodevelopmental Approach to Specific Learning Disorders: The Clinical Nature of the Problem.* London: MacKeith Press; 1998.

5. Missiuna C. Motor skill acquisition in children with developmental coordination disorder. *Adapt Phys Act Q.* 1994; 11(2), 214-235.

6. Geuze RH, Kalverboer AF. Inconsistency and adaptation in timing of clumsy children. *J Hum Movement Studies.* 1987; 13, 421-432.

7. Marchiori GE, Wall, AE, Bedingfield EW. Kinematic analysis of skill acquisition in physically awkward boys. *Adapt Phys Act Q.* 1987; 4, 305-315.

8. Van Dellen T, Geuze RH. Motor response processing in clumsy children. *J Child Psychol Psyc.* 1988; 29: 489-500.

9. Van Dellen T, Geuze RH. Experimental studies on motor control in clumsy children. In: Kalverboer AF, ed. *Developmental biopsychology: Experimental and observational studies of children at risk.* Ann Arbor, MI: University of Michigan Press; 1990.

10. Goodgold-Edwards SA, Cermak SA. Integrating motor control and motor learning concepts with neuropsychological perspectives on apraxia and developmental dyspraxia. *Am J Occup Ther.* 1990; 44, 431-438.

11. Vygotsky, L.S. Thinking and speech. In R.W. Reiber & A.S. Carton (Eds), The Collected Works of L.S. Vygotsky 1987; 39-28

12. Luria A, The directive function of speech in development. *Word.* 1959; 18, 341-352.

13. Luria A, *The role of speech in the regulations of normal and abnormal behaviors.* New York: Liveright; 1961.

14. Meichenbaum D. *Cognitive behaviour modification.* New York, NY: Plenum Press; 1977.

15. Meichenbaum D. *Cognitive behavior modification.* Workshop presented at Child and Parent Research Institute Symposium; London, Ontario, Canada. London, Ontario Canada; 1991.

16. Meichenbaum D. & Goodman, J. Training impulsive children to talk to themselves: a means of developing self-control. *J Abnorm Psych.*1971; 77, 115-126.

17. Feuerstein R, Rand Y. Mediated learning experience: An outline of the proximal etiology for differential development of cognitive functions. International Understanding, 1974; 9/10, 7-37.

18. Feuerstein R, Hoffman M, Jensen M, Tzuriel D, & Hoffman D. Learning to learn: Mediated learning experiences and instrumental enrichment. *Special Services in the Schools,* 1986, 3, 48-82.

19. Feuerstein R, Hoffman, M, Miller R. *Instrumental enrichment: An intervention program for cognitive modifiability.* Baltimore, MD: University Park Press; 1980.

20. Haywood H.C. A mediational teaching style. *The Thinking Teacher.* 1987; 4 (1), 1-6.

21. Haywood H.C. Bridging: A special technique of mediation. *The Thinking Teacher.* 1988; 4(4), 4-5.

22. Missiuna C, Malloy-Miller T, & Mandich A, Mediational techniques: Origins and application to occupational therapy in pediatrics. *Cdn J Occ Ther.* 1998; 65, 202-209.

23. Kamm K, Thelen E, & Jensen J.L. A dynamical systems approach to motor development. *Phys Ther.* 70, 763-775.

24. Bernstein N. *The coordination and regulation of movements.* London, Pergamon Press; 1967.

25. Schmidt R.A. A schema theory of discrete motor skill learning. *Psychol Rev,* 1975; 82, 225-260.

26. Schmidt R.A. *Motor control and learning: A behavioral emphasis.* Champaign, IL: Human Kinetics. 1988.

27. Thelen E, Kelso JA, Fogel A. Self-organizing systems and infant motor development. *Dev Rev.* 1987; 7,39-65.

28. Perry SB. Clinical implications of a dynamic systems theory. *Neurology Report.* 1998; 22, 4-10.

29. Eliasmith C. The third contender: A critical examination of the dynamicist theory of cognition. In: Thagard P, ed. *Mind readings: Introductory selections on cognitive science.* Cambridge, MA: MIT Press; 1998.

30. Burton AW, Miller DE. *Movement skill assessment.* Windsor, ON: Human Kinetics; 1998.

31. Thelen E. Motor development: A new synthesis. *Am Psychol,* 1995; 50, 79-95.

32. Gentile A.M. Implicit and explicit processes during acquisition of functional skills. *Scan J Occup Ther.* 1998; 5, 7-16.

33. Lee T.D., Swinnen S.P. & Serrien D.J. Cognitive effort and motor learning. *Quest,* 1994; 46, 328-344.

34. Canadian Association of Occupational Therapists. *Enabling occupation: An occupational therapy perspective.* Ottawa, ON: Author; 1997.

35. Law M, Cooper B, Strong S, Stewart D, Rigby P, & Letts L. The person-environment-occupation model: A transactive approach to occupational performance. *Can J Occup Ther* 1996; 57, 82-87.

36. Polatajko HJ. Naming and framing occupational therapy: A lecture dedicated to the life of Nancy B. *Can J Occup Ther.* 1992; 59, 189-200.

37. Polatajko HJ, Mandich A, Martini R. *Am J Occup Ther.* 2000.

38. Trombly C. Anticipating the future: Assessment of occupational function. *Am J Occup Ther,* 1993; 47, 253-257.

39. Van Sant AF. Motor control, motor learning and motor development. In: Montgomery PC, Connolly BH eds., Motor control and physical therapy. Hixson, TN: Chattanooga Group; 1991.

40. Mathiewitz V, Haugen JB. Evaluation of motor behavior: Traditional and contemporary views. In Trombly CA ed, *Occupational Therapy for physical dysfunction* (4th ed). Baltimore, MD: Williams and Wilkins; 1995.

41. Coster W. Occupation-centred assessment of children. *Am J Occup Ther.* 1998; 52, 337-344.

42. Bandura A. Self-efficacy: Toward a unifying theory of behavioral change. *Psychol Rev.* 1977; 84, 191-215. 1977; 84, 191-215.

43. Bandura A. Some reflections on reflections. *Psychological Inq.* 1990; 1, 101-105.

44. Bandura A. *Self-efficacy: The exercise of control.* New York: W.H. Freeman and Company; 1997.

45. Matherly T.A. Effects of prior success or failure on performance under varying goal conditions. *J Soc Behav Pers.* 1986; 1, 267-277.

46. Beery J.M, West R.L. Cognitive self-efficacy in relation to personal mastery and goal setting across the life span. *Int J Behav Dev.* 1993; 16, 351-379.

47. Pressley M, Forrest-Pressley DL, Elliott-Faust D, Miller G. Children's use of cognitive strategies: How to teach strategies and what to do if they can't be taught. In: Pressley M & Brainerd CJ eds., *Cognitive learning and memory in children: Progress in cognitive development research.* New York, NY: Springer-Verlag; 1985.

48. Pressley M, Snyder BL, Cariglia-Bull T. How can good strategy use be taught to children? Evaluation of six alternative approaches. In (ed.) *Transfer of learning.* Orlando, FL: Academic Press; 1987.

49. Borkowski JG, Carr M, Pressley M. Spontaneous strategy use: Perspectives from metacognitive theory. *Intelligence.* 1987; 11, 61-75.

50. Lenz BK, Ellis ES, Scanlon D. *Teaching learning strategies to adolescents and adults with learning disabilities.* Austin, TX: Pro-Ed;1996.

51. Kramer P, Hinojosa J. *Frames of reference for pediatric occupational therapy.* Philadelphia, PA: Lippincott Williams & Wilkins; 1999.

Cognitive Orientation
to Daily Occupational Performance
(CO-OP):
Part II–
The Evidence

Helene J. Polatajko
Angela D. Mandich
Linda T. Miller
Jennifer J. Macnab

SUMMARY. CO-OP is a child-centred, cognitive based intervention, focused on enabling children to achieve their functional goals. It has

Helene J. Polatajko, PhD, OT(C), is Professor and Chair, Department of Occupational Therapy, and Professor, Department of Rehabilitation Science, Faculty of Medicine, University of Toronto, Toronto, Ontario, Canada, and Professor, Faculty of Education, The University of Western Ontario, London, Ontario, Canada. Angela D. Mandich, MSc, OT(C), is a doctoral candidate, School of Kinesiology, and Instructor, School of Occupational Therapy, The University of Western Ontario, London, Ontario, Canada. Linda T. Miller, PhD, is Assistant Professor, School of Occupational Therapy, Faculty of Health Sciences, The University of Western Ontario. Jennifer J. Macnab, BA, PhD candidate, is affiliated with the Department of Epidemiology & Biostatistics, Faculty of Medicine, The University of Western Ontario, London, Ontario, Canada. All of the authors are members of the Developmental Coordination Disorder Research Group.

Address correspondence to: Helene J. Polatajko, PhD, OT(C), Department of Occupational Therapy, Faculty of Medicine, University of Toronto, 256 McCaul Street, Toronto, Ontario, Canada M5T 1W5 (E-mail: h.polatajko@utoronto.ca).

Funded by the Cloverleaf Charitable Foundation.

[Haworth co-indexing entry note]: "Cognitive Orientation to Daily Occupational Performance (CO-OP): Part II–The Evidence." Polatajko, Helene J. et al. Co-published simultaneously in *Physical & Occupational Therapy in Pediatrics* (The Haworth Press, Inc.) Vol. 20, No. 2/3, 2001, pp. 83-106; and: *Children with Developmental Coordination Disorder: Strategies for Success* (ed: Cheryl Missiuna) The Haworth Press, Inc., 2001, pp. 83-106. Single or multiple copies of this article are available for a fee from The Haworth Document Delivery Service [1-800-342-9678, 9:00 a.m. - 5:00 p.m. (EST). E-mail address: getinfo@haworthpressinc.com].

been developed over the last nine years through a series of systematic studies that have specified the treatment protocol and evaluated its effect. Initially CO-OP was explored in two series of single case experimental studies. Subsequently, an informal follow-up study and a detailed analysis of the video-taped sessions of the approach were completed. Based on information from these studies, the approach was refined, key features elucidated and the protocol was specified. Next, a pilot randomized clinical trial was completed. The trial was conducted to determine how best to approach a full scale randomized clinical trial on the effectiveness of CO-OP, relative to the current therapeutic approach. Finally, a retrospective chart audit was carried out to examine the cumulative evidence on the effectiveness of CO-OP in improving the performance of children with DCD. This paper presents a detailed summary of these five studies and discusses the implications of the findings. *[Article copies available for a fee from The Haworth Document Delivery Service: 1-800-342-9678. E-mail address: <getinfo@haworthpressinc.com> Website: <http://www.HaworthPress.com> © 2001 by The Haworth Press, Inc. All rights reserved.]*

KEYWORDS. Evidence-based practice, motor learning disability, cognitive intervention, DCD

School-based health professionals receive a large number of referrals for children who exhibit mild motor or sensory motor problems that interfere with their performance at school. Often these children exhibit problems of sufficient severity to warrant the diagnosis of Developmental Coordination Disorder (DCD). "The essential feature of Developmental Coordination Disorder is a marked impairment in the development of motor coordination . . . that significantly interferes with academic achievement or activities of daily living."[1] In the past, children with DCD were provided intensive treatment for extended periods of time in clinics or schools.[2-4] Recent cutbacks in funding have seriously reduced services to these children. The rationale provided for cutting services has included issues of large numbers, the high cost of treatment, relatively small treatment effects, and the presumed unimportance of the problem. However, contrary to previous beliefs that this is a benign childhood condition, it is now clear from longitudinal studies that the condition persists into adulthood[1] and that there can be serious long-term sequelae.[5-8] Children with DCD are at risk for increased reliance on educational, social, mental health, vocational and economic services as they develop. Effective management of this condition is, therefore, an important health issue.

The approach to the treatment of children with DCD, traditionally, has been based on sensory-motor (reflex-hierarchical) models of motor development which focus on decreasing motor impairment (see Mandich et al., this volume, for a discussion). For several reasons, these approaches, which stem from the 'therapeutic concept of rebuilding control of the motor system,' (p. 14)[9] are now being reexamined. First, studies investigating the effectiveness of these approaches, for the most part, have failed to demonstrate any significant effects due to treatment[10-13] with most investigators reporting small, or no treatment effects.[14-19] Second, contemporary literature on motor learning and control suggests that the reflex-hierarchical model does not adequately explain skill acquisition and performance. Rather, current theories of motor learning emphasize the importance of the interaction of the person, the task and the environment in skill acquisition. The focus of treatment, therefore, should be on task performance.[20-23] In keeping with this, a number of experts have suggested that cognitive, or problem-solving approaches, should be considered in the treatment of children with DCD.[24-27] Finally, as reflected in current practice,[2] therapists are searching for effective alternatives that are quicker and more portable than the traditional approaches.

In 1991, Polatajko and colleagues[28] began to search for a new approach to children with DCD. It was considered that Meichenbaum's cognitive behavioural[29,30] approach, based on verbal self instructional training, was promising because it focussed on skill building, had been used effectively with other children with similar difficulties, and was consistent with contemporary thoughts on motor learning. This new approach, called Cognitive Orientation to daily Occupational Performance (CO-OP), combines Meichenbaum's cognitive behavioural approach with a client-centred framework[31] and the mediational techniques of Feuerstein and colleagues.[32-34] The CO-OP approach is a highly individualized one in which children are guided in the use of a global problem-solving strategy and the identification of domain-specific strategies that will enable new and effective ways of achieving their individually chosen functional goals.

Over the past nine years, Polatajko and colleagues have undertaken a program of study designed to develop and evaluate CO-OP. Initially CO-OP was explored in two series of single case experimental studies. Because of the heterogeneity of the DCD population, it was determined that a single case experimental design was the research paradigm of choice for exploring the efficacy of this new treatment. Further, single case experimental design, with direct replication, is a good method for developing a new treatment protocol and initially evaluating a treatment effect.[35]

The first series of single case experimental studies (SCES), carried out by a single therapist, included 10 children.[36,37] This allowed for one original experiment and nine direct replications, exceeding the recommended number of replications.[35] It was felt important to have a large enough sample to conduct a preliminary investigation of the transferability of the effect. Thus, the first series of SCES included a within-group design component, using standardized measures of related behaviours, administered by an independent assessor.

Ottenbacher[38] pointed out that the generalizability of a treatment effect needs to be demonstrated across clients, settings, and therapists before a treatment can attain broad acceptance. Ottenbacher described three phases to establish the generalizability of SCES results. In phase one, several direct replications must be conducted to establish a potential treatment effect. This first phase of generalizability was satisfied by the successful single case experiment with one child and the direct replications with nine other children conducted by the therapist in the series one SCES.[36,37] The second phase of generalizability requires replication across, clients, settings and therapists. This was satisfied by Martini and Polatajko,[39-41] by conducting a systematic replication with four additional children. Subsequently, an informal follow-up study[42] and a detailed analysis of the video-taped sessions of Studies I and II[43-45] were completed. Based on the information from these studies, the approach was refined, key features were elucidated and the protocol was specified. Next, a pilot randomized clinical trial[46] was completed. The trial was conducted to determine how best to approach a full scale RCT on the effectiveness of CO-OP, relative to the current therapeutic approach. This satisfied Ottenbacher's third phase of generalizability, showing clinical replication of the treatment effect and also provided evidence of the effect of CO-OP as compared to current treatment practices. Finally, a retrospective chart audit was carried out to examine the cumulative evidence on the effectiveness of CO-OP in improving the performance of children with DCD. The purpose of this paper is to present a detailed summary of these five studies and to discuss the implications of the findings.

STUDY I:
SINGLE CASE EXPERIMENTS–
SERIES ONE AND WITHIN-GROUP STUDY

The use of a cognitive approach in the treatment of the performance problems of children with DCD, initially called Verbal Self Guidance (VSG), was first explored by Wilcox and Polatajko[36, 37] in a series of single case experiments. One original single case experiment and nine direct replications were carried out to determine if the global problem-solving strategy, adapted from Meichenbaum's[29, 30] cognitive behavioural approach, could be used to improve the performance of children with DCD. As well, a within-group design was used to examine skill acquisition and to explore skill transfer.

The specific research questions addressed were[36]:

Can children with DCD learn the global problem-solving strategy?
Can children with DCD use the global problem-solving strategy to acquire the skills to perform three activities of their choice?
Once learned, are the performance skills maintained?
Does performance improve in other areas?

The sample consisted of 10 children, 4 girls and 6 boys, referred to occupational therapy for motor problems, all of whom recently had been involved in a randomized clinical trial of the process oriented treatment approach.[16] Four had been in the control group in the previous study, three in the process oriented treatment group, and two in the traditional treatment group. All children met the DSM-IV[1] criteria consistent with a diagnosis of DCD, were between the aged of 7-12 years, were of normal intelligence, had normal or corrected vision and hearing, and were identified by an occupational therapist as exhibiting motor problems. Children with neurological disorders were excluded. The 10 children and their families volunteered to attend treatment during the summer.

The children participated in 13, 50 minute, one-to-one sessions (1 baseline, 10 treatment, 1 post treatment, and 1 follow-up, 12 weeks post treatment), all conducted by a single therapist. In the first session the COPM was used to help children identify the three skills they needed, wanted, or were expected to perform that were difficult for them. Children were videotaped performing each of the three tasks, repeatedly, for baseline purposes. An attempt was made to have at least three repetitions of each behaviour, where possible. No attempt was made to have more frequent repetitions for baseline as it was felt that it was inappropriate to ask a child to repeatedly demonstrate failure on an activity that has been identified by the child as something that he or she cannot perform. In the following session they were taught Meichenbaum's global problem solving strategy, goal-plan-do-check. This is a four-step, problem solving strategy that teaches children to identify a goal, to state their plan for achieving it, to do the activity and then to check how successful they were. Throughout the 10 treatment sessions, Meichenbaum's self-instruction training concepts were used and the children were actively encouraged to use the goal-plan-do-check strategy to verbally guide themselves in learning to perform the three skills they had chosen. A puppet, Mr. GoalPlan-DoCheck, was introduced to the children as the president of a detective club. The children were invited to become members and solve the performance mysteries of the skills they had chosen to learn. Parents were invited to be present throughout, either in the room or on the other side of a one-way mirror. All sessions were videotaped.

The outcome measures used for the single case experiment component of the study were based on behavioral observation. For each child-chosen skill, percentage of time actively spent on-task, duration of the task performance, and performance quality were recorded by the investigator, using the video taped recordings of the baseline session, the treatment sessions, the post-treatment probe session and the follow-up session. In order to rate performance quality operational definitions were created and a scale was designed to rate performance quality. In all, 30 operational definitions and task specific quality performance rating scales were created for the 30 skills chosen by the children (see Table 1). Criteria were established for successful performance of each activity. For example, for the activity "handwriting," the criteria for a given child might have been: writes on line, forms all letters properly, appropriate spacing between words, legible product. The performance rating scale was as follows: 0 = met no criteria; 1 = met some criteria, poor quality of performance and product; 2 = met most criteria, poor quality of performance and product; 3 = met most criteria, fair quality of performance and product; 4 = met all criteria, fair quality of performance and product; 5 = met all criteria, excellent quality of performance and product.

The standardized measures used for the within-group design were: the Canadian Occupational Performance Measure (COPM),[47] which addressed the issue of skill acquisition, and the Vineland Adaptive

TABLE 1. Study I and II: Activities Chosen by the Children

Child	Activity One	Activity Two	Activity Three
STUDY I			
1	shuffling playing cards	slicing cheese, tomatoes, buns	writing capital letters
2	baking "good for you" cookies	cutting meat and bread	writing faster, "with the need for fewer corrections"
3	applying nail polish	shampooing hair	printing, beginning writing
4	making a dragon kite	writing speed, legibility	making a bed
5	folding paper "straight"	cutting paper	forming and joining letters
6	performing a karate kata	using chopsticks	making french toast
7	making hamburgers	writing numbers	playing baseball
8	writing capital letters	pitching a slo-pitch ball	sewing with needle/thread
9	cutting food with cutlery	printing	catching small balls
10	alphanumeric keyboarding	running cross-country "better"	copying numbers from blackboard
STUDY II			
1	hitting hockey targets	printing capital and small letters	twirling spaghetti on a spoon
2	making ice cream	typing on computer	throwing basketball into net
3	performing a karate kata	running faster	cutting cucumbers
4	skipping rope	printing capital and small letters	making paper airplanes

Note: Quotation marks indicate child's description

Behaviour Scales (VABS),[48] the Developmental Test of Visual Motor Integration (VMI),[49] the Test of Motor Impairment (TOMI),[50] the Child Behavior Checklist/4-18,[51] and the Eyberg Child Behaviour Inventory,[52] which explored issues of generalization and transfer. All measures, except for the COPM, were administered by an independent assessor at baseline and at follow-up, 12 weeks post treatment. The COPM, which is considered as much a part of the intervention as an outcome measure, was administered by the therapist on three occasions: at baseline, post treatment, and at follow-up.

While it is beyond the scope of this paper to present all the results of this study, the more germane data are presented here, i.e., the results addressing skill acquisition and transfer to adaptive behaviour and performance.

Skill acquisition was addressed in the single case experiments. For child 1, the first participant in the study, the single case data showed an important increase in performance quality between baseline and follow-up, for all three activities. For two activities, the increase was greatest between baseline and post-treatment, for the third activity it was greatest between post-treatment and follow-up (see Figure 1). This effect was replicated across nine children. The data for eight of the other children were similar, showing improvements in performance quality over baseline for 23* of 24 activities. One child** made only small to moderate gains. In sum, the single case data showed that 10 out of 10 children improved their performance on their chosen activities and maintained their performance 12 weeks after the end of treatment. Nine out of the 10 children learned to meet all performance criteria for their chosen skills with fair or excellent quality and showed maintenance 12 weeks later. This held true across 29 out of the 30 activities chosen by the children.

The COPM[47] also addressed the question of skill acquisition, on a group basis. These data mirrored the observational data, providing validation of the observational data. The children, as a group, across all 30 activities, reported dramatic improvements in performance and satisfaction for their chosen activities. The group means rose from 2.2 and 2.5 on performance and satisfaction, respectively, at baseline, to

---

*One child met all performance criteria for one of his three chosen activities at baseline.

**This child did not attend the full number of sessions and attended sporadically for the sessions he did attend. He was not present for the post-treatment session, but was present for follow-up.

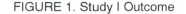

FIGURE 1. Study I Outcome

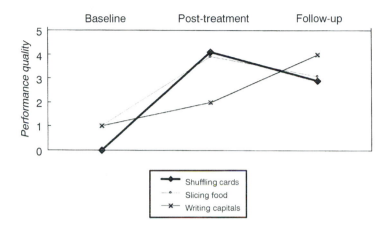

9.2 and 9.5, respectively, at post-treatment, to 8.7 and 8.9, respectively, at the 12 week follow-up (see Table 2). All differences between baseline and post-treatment and baseline and follow-up were significant. The differences between post-treatment and follow-up were not significant, indicating maintenance of the skills learned. Thus both the observational data and the COPM data indicated that the children learned to perform the three activities they had found difficult and maintained their skills 12 weeks post treatment.

Transfer of skills was explored using the COPM, VABS, VMI, and TOMI. The results for these were also promising. The VABS,[48] showed significant improvement, as the COPM had done. This indicates that the improvements in performance were not limited to the skills focused on in treatment. Transfer to specific motor skills, explored with the VMI,[49] and the TOMI,[50] is less clear. Changes, when they occurred, were in the expected direction, but the differences in scores between baseline and follow-up did not reach statistical significance. Given the limited power related to the small sample size, this result is difficult to interpret. It may indicate a lack of transfer or an inadequate sample size. Post hoc power analyses indicated an effect size (d) of .16 for the VMI, and .62 for the TOMI. By Cohen's criteria[53] these effect sizes are considered small and medium, respectively. For the VMI, this would suggest that the nonsignificant finding was due to a lack of transfer. In contrast, TOMI's data not reaching significance was probably due to insufficient sample size.

TABLE 2. Study I–Within-Group Outcomes (N = 10)

	Pre-test M *(SD)*	Post-test M *(SD)*	t Pre-Post	Follow-up M *(SD)*	t Pre-Follow-up
COPM⁺					
Performance	2.2 (1.6)	9.2 (1.4)	−17.07**	8.7 (1.8)	−14.46**
Satisfaction	2.5 (1.6)	9.5 (1.1)	−14.48**	8.9 (2.1)	−12.6**
VINELAND					
Composite	69.9 (10.6)			85.2 (14.6)	−5.18*
Communication	65.1 (12.0)			79.5 (18.6)	−3.38*
Daily Living Skills	81.6 (8.4)			90.4 (10.9)	−3.43*
Socialization	79.0 (14.4)			95.7 (14.3)	−6.69**
TEST OF VISUAL-MOTOR INTEGRATION (VMI)					
	84.3 (10.9)			81.9 (10.1)	0.52
TEST OF MOTOR IMPAIRMENT (TOMI)					
Total Raw Score	7.1 (3.5)			6.3 (2.4)	0.35
Manual dexterity	3.2 (2.0)			2.2 (1.9)	
Ball skills	1.0 (1.4)			1.2 (0.8)	
Balance	3.0 (1.2)			2.9 (1.1)	

*p < .05
**p < .01
+ COPM was administered on three occasions, the other measures were administered on two occasions.

92

To conclude, the results of series one were promising. The first single case experiment indicated that children with DCD could learn to use a global problem-solving strategy which could be used to acquire skills that are difficult for these children and that these skills are maintained. The nine direct replications showed that this was a reproducible effect and provided some evidence of skill transfer. Further development and testing of this cognitive approach was indicated.

STUDY II:
SYSTEMATIC REPLICATION

Martini[39-41] carried out a systematic replication of the single case experiment component of Study I. The purpose of Study II was to determine if the results obtained in Study I could be replicated by another therapist with four new children with DCD. Using a systematic replication approach, one original single case experiment and three replications were carried out, as recommended by Hersen and Barlow.[35] The basic research question addressed was:

> *With another therapist*, can children with DCD learn a global problem-solving strategy and use it to learn to perform three activities of their choice?

As in Study I, all children, one girl, three boys, met the DSM-IV criteria consistent with the diagnosis of DCD, were between the ages of 7-12 years, were of normal intelligence, had normal or corrected vision and hearing, and were identified by an occupational therapist as exhibiting features of DCD. Children with neurological disorders were excluded.

The measures used included the COPM,[47] the Performance Quality Rating Scale (PQRS),[39] a five-point behavioural observation scale used to rate the quality of activity performance, time on task, percentage correct use of the Goal-Plan-Do-Check (GPDC) strategy, and evidence of metacognition as reported by the children in response to questions probing strategy use. No attempts were made to address the question of maintenance and transfer in Study II.

The procedures used were the same as those in Study I with the addition of establishing inter-rater reliability for the behavioural observations. The therapist was trained in the cognitive approach by the authors of Study I. As no formal written treatment protocol existed, the therapists began training by reading about cognitive behaviour modification and viewing the videotapes of Study I and discussing key points. The therapist was video-taped and received supervision throughout the implementation of the approach.

The findings of Study I were replicated by the PQRS and COPM results (see Table 3). The children identified similar activities (see Table 1); learned the global strategy, used it to acquire their chosen skills, improved their performance and reported improved performance and satisfaction. Thus, the systematic replication was successful and provided evidence that the CO-OP approach was generalizable across therapists (see Martini & Polatajko, 1998, for a complete description[41]).

STUDY III:
INFORMAL FOLLOW-UP AND VIDEO TAPE ANALYSIS

Given the positive results of Studies I and II, it was decided to pursue the development of CO-OP. First, an informal follow-up with the children from Studies I and II was carried out.[42] Using an open-ended telephone questionnaire, an independent interviewer spoke with the parents of the children who had participated in Studies I and II. Parent reports indicated that the children continued to have the skills over the two or more years since their CO-OP treatment. Often there were also reports of continued improvement and further skill development. However, continued use of the strategy did not occur spontaneously. Thus it was decided to include a parent participation component in the approach.

Next, a detailed analysis of the video-taped sessions from Studies I and II was conducted to identify the salient strategies of the approach.[43-45] Analysis of 140 hours of this therapy provided verification of the use of the global strategy in skill acquisition and pointed to the identification of 8 domain specific strategies that supported specific skill acquisition. While the global strategy seemed necessary for skill acquisition, it seemed to be insufficient. Frequently, domain specific strategies were required to enable the child to carry out the task (for details, please see Mandich et al., this volume[45]). Thus, the global cognitive strategy Goal-Plan-Do-Check (GPDC) seemed to be acting as a framework for the identification of the domain specific strategies necessary to complete the task. This finding not only supported the use

TABLE 3. Study II–Systematic Replication Outcomes

		Baseline Activity			Post-treatment Activity		
		1	2	3	1	2	3
PQRS[1] mean score	Child 1	2.3	2.5	2.5	4.5	4.5	5
	Child 2	0	.17	1.7	3	1.3	3.7
	Child 3	0	2	3	4	3.7	4.8
	Child 4	0	2	0	4.8	3	3.7
COPM[2]							
Performance	Child 1	1	2	3	10	10	10
	Child 2	2	3	2	10	9	10
	Child 3	5	2	4	10	10	10
	Child 4	1	2	1	10	10	10
Satisfaction	Child 1	1	2	3	10	10	10
	Child 2	1	5	2	10	10	10
	Child 3	5	1	1	10	10	10
	Child 4	1	1	1	10	10	10

[1] PQRS, Performance Quality Rating Scale, is a five-point scale, where: 0 is no activity criteria are met, and 5 is all activity criteria are met with good quality.

[2] COPM, is a ten-point scale, where: 1 is low and 10 is high.

of the approach, but more importantly, allowed for the elucidation of the strategies being used and the specification of the treatment protocol. At this point, the treatment approach, and its name, were changed to reflect these new findings. Moving from Verbal Self Guidance (VSG) to Cognitive Orientation to daily Occupational Performance (CO-OP), both the global problem-solving strategy and domain specific strategies were incorporated into the treatment protocol.

STUDY IV:
CLINICAL REPLICATION–PILOT RCT

In 1998, Miller and Polatajko and colleagues carried out a pilot randomized clinical trial of CO-OP (see Miller et al.[48] for a detailed description). The objective of this pilot study was to determine the feasibility of a full scale RCT comparing CO-OP with the current treatment typically given to children with DCD. This study evaluated performance improvements on three tasks identified by the child as problematic and chosen by the child for the focus of treatment and generalization and transferability. The study was carried out using a random groups design with children randomly assigned to either the CO-OP or current treatment approach (CTA) groups. The current treatment approach is an eclectic combination of neuromuscular, multi-sensory, and biomechanical approaches.

Twenty children, six girls, 14 boys, between the ages of 7 and 12 (mean age of 9.05 years, *SD* = 1.23) participated in this study. All children had been referred to the university clinic for performance problems. All had normal intelligence, were identified by a therapist as having motor problems and met the DSM-IV criteria for DCD. All could identify three performance issues during administration of the COPM.

Three therapists, all experienced in working in the schools with children with motor problems. participated in the study: one, experienced with CO-OP, treated five children, using the CO-OP approach only; one, having no knowledge of CO-OP, treated five children using the CTA approach, only; and one, also with no a priori knowledge of CO-OP, used CTA with the first five children she saw, and then was trained in CO-OP for use with the next five children she saw. In both groups, the three treatment goals were child-chosen. In the CO-OP group, the treatment was carried out in the manner described in the protocol (see Polatajko et al.,[28] this volume). The children in the CTA group participated in the same number of sessions as those in the CO-OP group. The content of the CTA treatment was left entirely to the therapists; they were encouraged to do what ever they felt would get the best results. The treatments were monitored by observers who used pre-established criteria to verify that the CTA therapists were not using a problem solving approach.

The measures used to assess skill acquisition were: the COPM[47] and the PQRS, adapted to a 10-point scale from Martini's[39] original 5-point scale. Measures of adaptive behaviour, handwriting, general motor proficiency, and self-esteem were used to evaluate generalization and transfer. The measures used were: the VABS,[48] the Evaluation Tool of Children's Handwriting (ETCH), the Bruininks-Oseretsky Test of Motor Proficiency (BOTMP),[54] the VMI,[49] and the Self-Perception Profile for Children (SPPC),[55] respectively. All measures were administered pre and post treatment by an independent evaluator, blinded to group status, with one exception. The COPM, which, as indicated above, serves both as a component of the CO-OP approach and a pre-post measure, was administered by the treating therapist.

A series of two factor ANOVAs comparing the two treatment groups across pretest and post-test scores were used to analyze the data. Results indicated that both treatments lead to improved COPM self-ratings of performance and satisfaction. However, improvements in the CO-OP group were significantly greater than those in the CTA group. These results were paralleled by PQRS scores, and the Motor scores on the VABS, demonstrating that children in the CO-OP group were rated by independent observers and by standardized techniques to have improved significantly more than children in the CTA group.

In conclusion, self-report, blinded observer report, and standardized assessment results from an independent, blinded tester, all demonstrated the effectiveness of the CO-OP approach in this pilot study. This was a remarkable finding. The ability to detect significant group differences with a sample of only 10 children per group implies that the magnitude of the effect of CO-OP treatment was very large. Indeed, group differences found were in the order of one standard deviation and greater for the COPM and the PQRS, and approaching one standard deviation for the VABS domain scores. Effect sizes of this magnitude are rare, if not non-existent, in treatment studies with this population. The results of this study, in combination with the results of the single case studies reported previously, provide strong support for the use of CO-OP with this population.

STUDY V:
CLINICAL REPLICATION–CUMULATIVE EVIDENCE

CO-OP has now been used in the university clinic for approximately six years. Four therapists have been trained in the approach and have used it with 35 children for 105 performance goals that they identified as things they want to, need to, or were expected to do. The children all were between the ages of seven and twelve and attended the university clinic on evenings or weekends. At least one parent for each child was present for a minimum of four of the sessions.

As a matter of routine, unless the data are already available on the child's chart from elsewhere, the treating therapist does the intake assessments, to verify that the child meets the criteria for DCD and is appropriate for the CO-OP approach. The intake assessments include the Kaufman Brief Intelligence Test (K-BIT),[56] the Movement Assessment Battery for Children (M-ABC),[57] and the VMI.[49] The therapist also administers the COPM,[47] at the outset of treatment to establish the child's goals and then at the end of treatment to measure outcome. Where resources permit, an independent tester is used to administer outcome measures, pre and post treatment, to provide independent validation of goal attainment and address generalizability and transferability. The former is done by applying the PQRS[39] to videotaped sessions. The latter is done Using the survey form of the interview edition of the VABS.[48] From time to time these measures are changed, e.g., at times the M-ABC is used as a pre and post measure, while at other times (e.g., during the pilot RCT, see above) it is used only as an intake measure.

For Study V, the data from these measures were compiled in a retrospective chart audit of clinic records to determine the clinical replicability of CO-OP. Specifically, an analysis of data from a retrospective chart audit was completed to determine if the treatment effects reported in Studies I and II could be replicated in a clinic by different therapists working with different children with DCD.

The retrospective chart audit yielded data for 25 of 35 children (10 children were excluded from the analyses because of missing data). All 25 children met the criteria for DCD and many (40%) also had other diagnoses, e.g., learning disabilities or attention deficit disorder. The measures for which data were available appear in Table 4, as do the sample sizes associated with each measure. As can be seen, typical of any retrospective chart audit, there were many missing data. This occurred for several reasons, some of which are alluded to above, i.e., feasibility, data on like measures available from other sources and studies requiring different measures. Using a within group design, the data were analyzed to determine pre/post test differences. Paired t-tests were carried out. The results (see Table 4) show that CO-OP positively affects direct skill acquisition. This can be seen in the significant improvement in the COPM scores on both performance and satisfaction. The results also indicate that the effects of CO-OP generalize and transfer. This can be seen in the significant improvement on the M-ABC in the areas of ball skills, balance and overall performance; on the VMI; and on the VABS in the areas of communication and motor performance and on the composite. Because of the relatively small overall sample size, the t-test analyses were performed without error rate control for multiple analyses. However, application of a Bonferroni adjustment* does not alter the interpretation of the analyses, indicating that, even in the context of a very conservative adjustment to the Type 1 error rate, several important effects are apparent. Most notably, the M-ABC Total Impairment Score, the VABS Composite Score, and the Performance and Satisfaction scores of the COPM all yield significant treatment effects.

When considered in combination with the relatively small sample size of some of the t-tests performed, the conservative treatment of significance levels, the effects are considerable. Thus, the results of Study V provide evidence of the clinical replicability of the treatment effect first observed in Study I.

DISCUSSION

The purpose of this paper was to present a summary of a series of studies carried out in the development and evaluation of a new treatment

---

*Given the number of t-tests performed, it is statistically possible that some of the effects found represent Type 1 errors. To control for this, a Bonferroni adjustment was made to the Type 1 error rate by dividing alpha across the 16 t-tests performed (a = .05/16 = .003). This adjustment yields a conservative interpretation of the t-test results.[58]

TABLE 4. Study V–Clinical Replication Outcomes

	N	Mean		SD		t	df	p value
		Pre	Post	Pre	Post			
COPM Performance	25	3.49	8.32	1.56	1.35	11.68	24	< .001
Satisfaction		3.59	9.21	1.72	0.83	14.07	24	<.001
M-ABC Manual Dexterity[1]	14	7.39	6.68	4.46	3.93	0.97	13	.349
Ball Skills		3.21	1.93	3.12	2.79	2.49	13	.027
Balance		6.11	3.18	4.09	3.92	3.07	13	.009
Total Impairment		16.71	11.78	8.94	8.78	3.95	13	.002
VMI	24	92.08	98.33	14.47	13.44	2.74	23	.012
VABS Communication	15	88.87	97.80	13.95	13.95	3.02	14	.009
Daily Living Skills		83.33	88.53	16.28	13.34	2.09	14	.055
Socialization		86.13	90.73	15.25	13.39	1.86	14	.085
Motor		87.47	100.20	19.88	16.26	2.94	14	.011
Composite		83.20	90.13	13.85	14.58	4.16	14	.001

[1] The M-ABC yields an impairment score, a decrease in score therefore indicates improvement.

approach to DCD and to discuss the implications of the finding. The approach, CO-OP, is adapted from Meichenbaum's cognitive behavioural approach and thus represents a very different perspective on motor skill acquisition and the performance problems of children with DCD. In contrast to traditional views, CO-OP is based on the premise that motor performance is not primarily an issue of neuromaturation, rather an issue of learning and that children with DCD have a motor learning problem. The series of five studies presented here have each, in a systematic fashion, contributed to an evaluation of this basic premise and the development of a new treatment approach with demonstrated effectiveness.

The potential of a learning model to guide the skill acquisition of children with a mild motor impairment was first demonstrated in the series of single case experiments of Study I. Those findings indicated that strategy use, by itself, could enable a child with DCD to perform a difficult motor based activity, competently. This suggests that the performance issue is less likely a neuromaturational one and more likely one of learning. However, as Ottenbacher[38] pointed out, showing an effect at one time, with one therapist, is insufficient evidence to establish the efficacy of an approach. "The ultimate test of generalizability for any treatment finding is whether other therapists can implement the intervention procedure under other situational conditions with other clients and achieve similar outcomes" (p. 207).

Studies II, IV and V addressed the generalizability by demonstrating that the effect was reproducible across therapists, children and a large variety of activities. Study IV also showed that the approach was more effective than the current approach being used by experienced therapists. This not only satisfied Ottenbacher's third phase of generalizability, showing clinical replication of the treatment effect, it also provided evidence of the effect of CO-OP as compared to current treatment practices. Studies IV and V, together showed that the effect was not restricted to the skills directly considered in the course of treatment but also generalized and transferred to other related skills. Taken together these studies provide strong convergent evidence that CO-OP is an effective approach for use with children with DCD.

The outcome of this series of studies is not only a new treatment approach but also new insights into DCD and motor acquisition. Children with DCD comprise a significant proportion of school-aged children and studies have provided evidence suggesting that the long-term effects of this disorder are handicapping for these children. The program of research described here has identified a treatment approach that intervenes at the level of disability to improve performance in daily occupations. The approach in no way attempts to 'cure' DCD. There is, at present, no evidence that the impairment of motor coordination in these children can be cured. Indeed the success of this approach, embedded in a learning paradigm, in enabling children with DCD to use strategies to effect a change in performance, would suggest that this is not a problem in search of a cure. Rather, it is a problem in search of effective learning strategies that will enable the children to perform the activities they need to, want to, or are required to perform.

Consistent with the present health care trend of client-centred practice and consumer satisfaction, the CO-OP treatment approach actively involves the family. The approach is both cost effective, as evidenced by maintenance of acquired skills, and portable. CO-OP is a child-centred, cognitive based intervention, focused on enabling children to achieve their functional goals. It was developed to help children with DCD acquire functional skills that they find difficult to perform. CO-OP intervention is individually tailored and highly responsive to each child. The CO-OP approach builds upon the child's strengths and enables the child to improve his/her performance on self-selected activities. There is evidence that CO-OP is effective in enabling skill acquisition and there is growing indication that CO-OP also results in generalization and transfer of skills. The next step would be to evaluate the effectiveness of CO-OP when administered within the school setting, as opposed to the clinic setting.

ACKNOWLEDGEMENTS

The authors wish to acknowledge the important contributions of four groups to this work. First, we wish to express our gratitude to the three graduate students who devoted their thesis work to this endeavor. Anne Wilcox was visionary enough to take an idea and translate it into action. She pioneered the successful application of cognitive strategies to skill acquisition among children with mild motor problems. Rose Martini was courageous enough to hold herself up as the therapist who would replicate the results. She undertook to master this new technique and carry out a systematic replication. In doing so, she not only demonstrated that further development of the approach was warranted, but also how the approach could be taught to other therapists. Angie Mandich was insightful enough to question the assertions about the potency of the global strategy and searched for evidence of other strategy use. Angie's data provided evidence that the global strategy was a necessary component of the approach but not sufficient; that other strategies, specifically, domain specific strategies were important to skill acquisition. Second, our appreciation goes to the therapists who were willing to come to work in our research clinic to learn the approach: Katherine Harris, Becky Lawson, Leala Lee, Penny Letheren, and Viola Sternberger. Their thoughtful participation contributed to the refinement and elucidation of the key features of the approach. Third, we wish to acknowledge the contributions of the many children and their families who participated. We are truly indebted to them for raising the issues and guiding us in the discovery of a solution. Finally, we wish to thank our funders, the Hospital for Sick Children Foundation for funding the pilot RCT and the Cloverleaf Charitable Foundation which has been with us almost from the outset. Their continued interest in our work and their ongoing financial support have made this work possible.

REFERENCES

1. American Psychiatric Association. Motor skill disorder 315.40 Developmental coordination disorder. In *Diagnostic and statistical manual of mental disorders* (4th Ed.), (pp. 53-55) Washington, DC: American Psychiatric Association; 1994.

2. Mandich AD, Polatajko HJ, Macnab JJ, Miller LT. Treatment of children with Developmental Coordination Disorder: What is the evidence? *Phys Occup Ther Ped.* 2001; 20(2/3), 51-68.

3. Wallen M, Walker R. Occupational therapy practice with children with perceptual motor dysfunction: findings of a literature review and survey. *Aust Occup Ther J.* 1995; 42,15-25.

4. Yack E. Sensory integration: A survey of its use in the clinical setting. *Can J Occup Ther.* 1989; 56,229-235.

5. Cantell MH, Smyth MM, Ahonen TP. Clumsiness in adolescence: Educational, motor, and social outcomes of motor delay detected at 5 years. Special Issue: Developmental coordination disorder. *Adap Phys Acti Q.* 1994; 11, 129.

6. Henderson, SE. The natural history and long term consequences of clumsiness in children. *Proceedings of children and clumsiness: A disability in search of a definition.* October 11-14; 1994.

7. Kadesjo B, Gillberg C. Developmental coordination disorder in Swedish 7-year-old children. *J Am Acad Child Adoles Psychiat.* 1999; 38,820-828.

8. Schoemaker MM, Kalverboer AF. Social and affective problems of children who are clumsy: How early do they begin? *Adap Phys Acti Q.* 1994; 11,130-140.

9. Van Sant. Motor control, motor learning and motor development. In PC Montgomery, BH Connolly, (Eds.) *Motor control and physical therapy.* (pp. 13-28). Hixson, TN: Chatanooga Group; 1991.

10. Hoehn TP, Baumeister AA. A critique of the application of sensory integration therapy to children with learning disabilities. *J Learn Disabil.* 1994; 27,338-350.

11. Polatajko HJ, Kaplan BJ, Wilson B. Sensory integration treatment for children with learning disabilities: Its status 20 years later. *Occup Ther J Res.* 1992; 12, 323-341.

12. Polatajko HJ. The treatment of children with mild motor difficulties in OT: What do we know now? (Abstract). *Proceedings of 11th International Congress of the World Federation of Occupational Therapists*, London, England 1994; 856-858.

13. Kavale K, Mattson PD. One jumped off the balance beam: Metaanalysis of perceptualmotor training. *J Learn Disabil.* 1983; 16,165-173.

14. Kaplan BJ, Polatajko HJ, Wilson BN, Faris PD. Reexamination of sensory integration treatment: a combination of two efficacy studies. *J Learn Disabil.* 1993; 26, 342-347.

15. Polatajko, H. J., Law, M., Miller, J., Schaffer, R., Macnab, J. J. The effect of a sensory integration program on academic achievement, motor performance and self-esteem in children identified as learning disabled: Results of a clinical trial. *Occup Ther J Res.* 1991; 11,155-176.

16. Polatajko HJ, Macnab JJ, Anstett B, Malloy-Miller T, Murphy K, Noh S. A clinical trial of the process-oriented treatment approach for children with developmental co-ordination disorder. *Dev Med Child Neurol.* 1995; 37, 260-269.

17. Wilson B, Kaplan BJ, Fellowes S, Gruchy C, Faris P. The efficacy of sensory integration treatment compared to tutoring. *Phys Occup Ther Ped.* 1992; 12, 1-36.

18. Humphries T, Wright M, Mcdougall B, Vertes J. The efficacy of sensory integration therapy for children with learning disability. *Phys Occup Ther Ped.* 1990; 10, 1-17.

19. Humphries T, Wright M, Snider L, Mcdougall B. A comparison of the effectiveness of sensory integration therapy and perceptual motor training in treating children with learning disabilities. *J Develop Behav Pediatr.* 1992; 13,31-40.

20. Mathiowetz V, Haugen JB. Evaluation of motor behavior: Traditional and contemporary views. In CA Trombly, (Ed.), *Occupational therapy for physical dysfunction* (4th Ed.), (pp. 157-185) Baltimore: Williams and Wilkins; 1995.

21. Schmidt M. *Motor control and learning: A behavioral emphasis.* Champaign, IL, Human Kinetics Publishers; 1988.

22. Shumway-Cook A, Woollacott M. *Motor control: Theory and practical application.* Baltimore, ML: Williams & Wilkins; 1995.

23. Mulder T, Geurts S. The assessment of motor dysfunctions: Preliminaries to a disability-oriented approach. *Hum Mov Sci.* 1991; 10,565-574.

24. Bouffard M, Wall AE. A problem solving approach to movement skill acquisition: Implications for special populations. In G Reid, (Ed.), *Problems in Movement Control.* (pp. 107-131) North-Holland: Elsevier Science Publishers B.V.; 1990.

25. Goodgold-Edwards SA, Cermak SA. Integrating motor control and motor learning concepts with neuropsychological perspectives on apraxia and developmental dyspraxia. *Am J Occup Ther.* 1990; 44,431-439.

26. Henderson SE. Problems of motor development: Some practical issues. In BK Keogh, (Ed.), *Advances in Special Education, Volume 5.* (pp. 187-218) Greenwich, Conn.: JAI Press Inc.; 1986.

27. Sellers JS. Clumsiness: review of causes, treatments, and outlook. *Phys Occup Ther Ped.* 1995; 39-55.

28. Polatajko HJ, Mandich A, Missiuna C, Miller LT, Macnab JJ, Malloy-Miller T, Kinsella EA. Cognitive orientation to daily occupational performance (CO-OP): Part III–The protocol in brief. *Phys Occup Ther Ped.* 2001; 20(2/3), 107-123.

29. Meichenbaum D. *Cognitive-behavior modification: An integrative approach.* New York: Plenum Press; 1977.

30. Meichenbaum, D. *Cognitive-behavior modification: Workshop presented at the Child and Parent Research Institute symposium*; 1991.

31. Canadian Association of Occupational Therapists. *Enabling Occupation: An occupational therapy perspective.* Ottawa, ON: CAOT Publications ACE; 1997.

32. Feuerstein R, Haywood HC, Rand Y, Hoffman MB, Jensen MR. *Learning potential assessment device (L.P.A.D.) manual.* Jerusalem: Hadassah Wizo Canada Research Institute; 1986.

33. Haywood HC. A mediational teaching style. *The Thinking Teacher.* 1987; 4, 1-7.

34. Missiuna C, Malloy-Miller T, Mandich A. Mediational techniques: Origins and application to occupational therapy in paediatrics. *Can J Occup Ther.* 1998; 65, 202-209.

35. Hersen M, Barlow DH. *Single case experimental design: Strategies for studying behaviour change.* New York, NY: Pergamon Press; 1976.

36. Wilcox, A. L. Verbal self-guidance: An exploratory study with children with developmental coordination disorder. Unpublished master's thesis, The University of Western Ontario, London, ON Canada; 1994.

37. Wilcox A. Polatajko HJ. Verbal self-guidance as a treatment technique for children with developmental coordination disorder. (Abstract). *Can J Occup Ther.* 1993; Supplement: 20-20.

38. Ottenbacher KJ. Statistical analysis of single system data. In *Evaluating clinical change: strategies for occupational and physical therapists* (pp. 167-195) Baltimore: Williams and Wilkins; 1986.

39. Martini, R. Verbal self-guidance as an approach to the treatment of children with developmental coordination disorder: A systematic replication study. Unpublished master's thesis, The University of Western Ontario, London, ON Canada., 1994.

40. Martini R, Polatajko HJ. Verbal self-guidance in the treatment of children with developmental coordination disorder: A systematic replication study. (Abstract). *Can J Occup Ther.* 1995; 62:11.

41. Martini R, Polatajko HJ. Verbal self-guidance as a treatment approach for children with developmental coordination disorder: A systematic replication study. *Occup Ther J Res.* 1998; 18, 157-181.

42. Polatajko HJ, Mandich A, Martini R. CO-OP: Learning from follow-up data. (Abstract). *Can J Occup Ther* 1997; Suppl. 25.

43. Mandich, A. Cognitive Strategies and Motor Performance of Children with Developmental Coordination Disorder. Unpublished master's thesis, The University of Western Ontario, London, ON Canada, 1997.

44. Mandich, A., Polatajko, H. J., Miller, L. T., Macnab, J. J., and Missiuna, C. Cognitive strategies: Getting DCD kids to succeed. *From research to diagnostics and intervention, 4th biennial workshop on children with developmental coordination disorder.* Groningen, The Netherlands; October 7 and 8, 1999.

45. Mandich AD, Polatajko HJ, Missiuna C, Miller LT. Cognitive strategies and motor performance in children with Developmental Coordination Disorder. *Phys Occup Ther Ped.*; 2001; 20(2/3), 125-143.

46. Miller LT, Polatajko HJ, Missiuna C, Mandich A, and Macnab JJ. A Pilot Trial of a Cognitive Treatment for Children With Developmental Coordination Disorder. *Hum Mov Sci.* (accepted, 2000).

47. Law M, Baptiste S, Carswell-Opzoomer A, McColl MA, Polatajko NJ, Pollock N. *Canadian Occupational Performance Measure.* Toronto, ON: CAOT Publications ACE; 1991.

48. Sparrow SS, Balla DA, Cichetti DV. *Vineland Adaptive Behavior Scales:* Interview edition, expanded form manual. Circle Pines, MN: American Guidance Service; 1984.

49. Beery KA. *Developmental Test of Visual-Motor Integration.* (Rev. Ed.). Chicago: Follett; 1989.

50. Stott DH, Moyes FA, Henderson SE. *Test of Motor Impairment.* Guelph: Brook Educational Publishing Ltd; 1984.

51. Achenbach TM. *Manual for the child behavior checklist/4-18 and 1991 profile.* Burlington, VT: University of Vermont Department of Psychiatry; 1991.

52. Robinson EA, Eyberg SM, Ross AW. The standardization of an inventory of child conduct problem behaviors. *J Clin Child Psych.* 1980; 9,22-29.

53. Cohen J. *Statistical power analysis for the behavioral sciences.* (2nd Ed.). Hillsdale, NJ: L. Erlbaum Associates; 1988.

54. Bruininks RH. Bruininks-Oseretsky Test of Motor Proficiency. Minnesota: American Guidance Service; 1978.

55. Harter S. *Self perception profile for children.* Denver, CO: University of Denver (Department of Psychiatry); 1985.

56. Kaufman AS, Kaufman NL. *Kaufman brief intelligence test.* Circle Pines, MN: American Guidance Service; 1990.

57. Henderson SE, Sugden DA. *Movement Assessment Battery for Children (manual).* Kent, UK: The Psychological Corporation; 1992.

58. Keppel G. *Design and analysis: A researcher's handbook.* (3rd Ed.). Englewood Cliffs, NJ: Prentice Hall; 1991.

Cognitive Orientation
to Daily Occupational Performance
(CO-OP):
Part III–
The Protocol in Brief

Helene J. Polatajko
Angela D. Mandich
Cheryl Missiuna
Linda T. Miller
Jennifer J. Macnab
Theresa Malloy-Miller
Elizabeth A. Kinsella

Helene J. Polatajko, PhD, OT(C), is Professor and Chair, Department of Occupational Therapy; Professor, Department of Rehabilitation Science, Faculty of Medicine, University of Toronto, Toronto, Ontario, Canada; and Professor, Faculty of Education, The University of Western Ontario, London, Ontario, Canada. Angela D. Mandich, MSc, OT(C) is doctoral candidate, School of Kinesiology, and Instructor, School of Occupational Therapy, The University of Western Ontario. Cheryl Missiuna, PhD, OT(C) is Assistant Professor, School of Rehabilitation Science, and Co-Investigator, CanChild Centre for Childhood Disability Research, McMaster University, Hamilton, Ontario, Canada. Linda T. Miller, PhD, is Assistant Professor, School of Occupational Therapy, Faculty of Health Sciences, The University of Western Ontario. Jennifer J. Macnab, BA, is a doctoral candidate, Department of Epidemiology & Biostatistics, Faculty of Medicine, The University of Western Ontario. Theresa Malloy-Miller, MSc, OT(C), is Occupational Therapist, Thames Valley Children Centre, London, Ontario, Canada. All of the above authors are members of the Developmental Coordination Disorder Research Group. Elizabeth A. Kinsella, MAEd, OT(C) is doctoral candidate, Faculty of Education, The University of Western Ontario.

Address correspondence to: Helene J. Polatajko, PhD, OT(C), Department of Occupational Therapy, Faculty of Medicine, University of Toronto, 256 McCaul Street, Toronto, Ontario, Canada, M5T 1W5 (E-mail: h.polatajko@utoronto.ca).

[Haworth co-indexing entry note]: "Cognitive Orientation to Daily Occupational Performance (CO-OP): Part III–The Protocol in Brief." Polatajko, Helene J. et al. Co-published simultaneously in *Physical & Occupational Therapy in Pediatrics* (The Haworth Press, Inc.) Vol. 20, No. 2/3, 2001, pp. 107-123; and: *Children with Developmental Coordination Disorder: Strategies for Success* (ed: Cheryl Missiuna) The Haworth Press, Inc., 2001, pp. 107-123. Single or multiple copies of this article are available for a fee from The Haworth Document Delivery Service [1-800-342-9678, 9:00 a.m. - 5:00 p.m. (EST). E-mail address: getinfo@haworthpressinc.com].

SUMMARY. Parts I and II of this series introduced the Cognitive Orientation to daily Occupational Performance (CO-OP), a new approach to intervention that is based on the premise that cognition plays an important role in the acquisition of occupational skills and the development of occupational competency. Developed for use with children who have occupational performance deficits, CO-OP is an individualized, client-centred approach focused on strategy-based skill acquisition. This third paper in this series presents a brief description of the actual CO-OP protocol including its objectives, prerequisites and key features. *[Article copies available for a fee from The Haworth Document Delivery Service: 1-800-342-9678. E-mail address: <getinfo@haworthpressinc. com> Website: <http://www.HaworthPress.com> © 2001 by The Haworth Press, Inc. All rights reserved.]*

KEYWORDS. Cognitive approach, intervention, DCD, CO-OP

Cognitive Orientation to daily Occupational Performance (CO-OP) is an approach to intervention that uses the power of cognition to drive successful performance. The CO-OP approach is based on the premise that cognition plays an important role in the acquisition of occupational skills and, by extension, the development of occupational competency. Created for use with children who have occupational performance deficits, the CO-OP approach can be used to promote the acquisition of new skills and the improvement of existing skills. In CO-OP, intervention focuses on the use of cognitive strategies to solve performance problems and to develop occupational competency.

CO-OP developed as an intervention approach as a result of research being performed with children with Developmental Coordination Disorder (DCD).* These children (see Polatajko[1] for a description) appear to have difficulty with the motor aspects of performance, particularly when a novel motor task is to be performed. Traditionally, therapy for these children has focused on reducing the underlying motor impairment (see Mandich, Polatajko, Macnab, & Miller, this volume, for a description[2]). These approaches, based on sensory-motor (reflex-hierarchical) models of motor development, conceptualize

---

*Although to date CO-OP has only been formally investigated with children with DCD. Early experience with other clients suggests that, like other cognitive approaches, CO-OP is likely to have applications with other populations.

the motor performance problems of these children as stemming from some form of sensory, sensory-motor or sensory-integrative deficit and treatment is designed to ameliorate these underlying deficits. For the most part, these are physical approaches. During treatment, the child is actively engaged in a large variety of activities, often developmentally sequenced, that provide the sensory, sensory-motor, or sensory integrative experiences that are considered to be fundamental to motor performance. The assumption is that exposure to such activities will foster the development of these fundamental skills and consequently improve motor performance.[3]

CO-OP represents a different orientation to this traditional approach. In contrast with traditional approaches, CO-OP treatment is focused directly on occupational performance issues and is a verbal approach. During treatment, the child is actively engaged in solving performance problems and testing out solutions. The assumption is that performance is the result of the interaction between the child, the environment, and the occupation[4] and that cognitive strategies can be used to drive performance.[5]

CO-OP was developed in response to a need for an alternative to the established approaches to the treatment of children with DCD. For the most part, the more traditional approaches were quite costly and time-consuming, with treatments being lengthy and progress being slow. As well, there was mounting evidence that they were relatively ineffective.[2] Based on the results of a treatment outcome study in which the only positive effect found was for a direct skill-teaching task,[6] it was hypothesized that DCD was essentially a motor learning disability and that treatment should be approached from a skill acquisition or learning perspective, rather than a neuro-developmental perspective.[7]

The learning literature, in particular the cognitive behavior modification literature, was examined in search of a new approach to the treatment of the performance problems of children with DCD. As well, the contemporary motor literature was searched for a potential model of motor performance. Both bodies of literature supported the exploration of an approach embedded in a learning paradigm. The cognitive behavioral literature, particularly the work of Meichenbaum,[8] provided a potential framework. Verbal self-instruction, using the global problem solving strategy used by Meichenbaum in his cognitive behavioral approach was adopted as a cornerstone for the new approach. This was augmented by the mediational techniques of

Feuerstein and colleagues.[9,10] Finally the principles of client-centred practice espoused by the Canadian Association of Occupational Therapists[11] were embedded throughout. The result was the development of a new, child-centred, cognitive oriented approach to enabling occupational performance, called Cognitive Orientation to daily Occupational Performance, "CO-OP," for short.

CO-OP has been under development since 1991. The initial version, called Verbal Self-Guidance (VSG),[12,13] stressed the verbal guidance aspect of the approach. Results of this original study were promising so it was decided to continue to develop and test the approach. Martini[14-16] demonstrated that the results could be replicated with a different therapist. Closer examination of the approach by Mandich[17,18] showed that verbal self-guidance was only one of the features of this approach; that there were a number of additional cognitive strategies used throughout the therapy. To emphasize the importance of cognitive strategies, the name was changed to CO-OP.

Continued use of the CO-OP approach, within a research paradigm, has reinforced the original findings and provided evidence of the effectiveness of the approach, with numerous children, across several therapists.[19] Experience with the training of therapists in the CO-OP approach has resulted in the elucidation of the key features of this approach and has allowed for the refinement of the treatment protocol. What is presented in this third paper in the series, is a brief description of this protocol–it is beyond the scope of this paper to present a full, in depth description of the protocol.*

THE CO-OP APPROACH IN BRIEF

Cognitive Orientation to daily Occupational Performance (CO-OP) is an individualized, client-centred approach focused on strategy-based skill acquisition. CO-OP is essentially a cognitive approach to solving daily occupational performance problems. While acknowledging that occupational performance is a complex multivariate phenomenon resulting from the interaction of person, environment and

---

*The reader is cautioned that, in the experience of the authors, a written description of the approach appears to be insufficient to allow for its proficient use. Experience with training therapists has highlighted the extent to which this approach represents a deviation from traditional perspectives and, therefore, requires hands-on-training.

occupation,[11,20-28] the CO-OP approach focuses on the primacy of cognition and strategy use in skill acquisition and the development of occupational competency. In CO-OP, a global problem-solving strategy is used to frame the development of domain specific strategies that enable successful task performance and promote skill acquisition. CO-OP is a highly verbal approach in which cognitive strategies are mapped onto performance to facilitate and support performance.

Objectives

CO-OP has three basic objectives:

- *Skill acquisition:* the child learns to perform the required or desired skills. In CO-OP, a client-centred approach is used to identify the skills to be learned. *The Canadian Occupational Performance Measure* (COPM)[24] is used with the child to identify the three skills that he/she needs to, wants to, or is expected to do at school, home, or play that will be the focus of treatment. The COPM is a self-report measure that allows children to rate both their level of performance and satisfaction when carrying out tasks that they need to do on a regular basis.
- *Cognitive strategy development:* the child learns to use a global problem solving strategy to frame the discovery of domain specific strategies that will solve performance problems and thereby, improve performance and promote skill acquisition.
- *Generalization and transfer:* the child uses the newly acquired skills and strategies beyond the treatment session, in everyday life, and these skills and strategies serve as a foundation for learning related skills and strategies.

Prerequisites

For the CO-OP approach to be successful, there are a number of prerequisites for all involved: the child, his/her parents and/or caregivers and the therapist.

To benefit from the CO-OP approach, the child must:

- have sufficient cognitive and language ability to respond to the COPM;
- be able to identify three occupational goals;
- be able to respond and attend to the therapist;

- have the potential to perform the task; and
- have the motivation to learn three skills.

The approach is most successful if the parents and/or caregivers are involved and committed to implementing the approach beyond the treatment arena. Prior to beginning the intervention, it is ideal if therapists develop a partnership with parents, such that parents are committed to participating in the therapy sessions and to implementing CO-OP at home. It is important that parents understand the role that they play in helping their child acquire skills, develop cognitive strategies, and transfer and generalize these into everyday life.

To be able to implement the CO-OP approach successfully, the therapist must already bring with him or her effective communication skills, experience with the management of children with disabilities in a child-centered framework, excellent skills in task analysis, and a commitment to working with parents. In addition, the therapist must become proficient in the CO-OP approach.

KEY FEATURES OF THE CO-OP APPROACH

There are six key features to the CO-OP approach: session structure, child-chosen goals, dynamic performance analysis, cognitive strategies, enabling principles and parent/caregiver involvement (see Figure 1). Each is briefly described.

FIGURE 1. Key Features of CO-OP

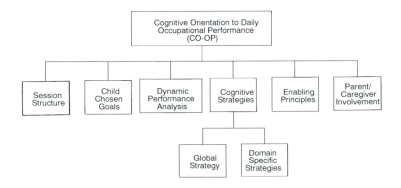

Session Structure

In Cognitive Orientation to daily Occupational Performance (CO-OP) the therapy sessions are offered according to a structured format (see Figure 2). CO-OP is usually delivered over twelve, one-to-one sessions, each of approximately one hour in length. Parents and/or caregivers are encouraged to observe as frequently as possible, in order to encourage generalization and transfer. The therapy process is divided into five phases: Preparation, Assessment, Introduction, Acquisition and Consolidation.

Child-Chosen Goals

CO-OP is a child-centred approach. The child's perspective is of central importance throughout, beginning with the process of goal setting and continuing throughout the intervention. A child-centered approach is used for several reasons. First it is consistent with a general trend in health care recognizing that children should have a voice in the interventions that concern them[29-31] and second it is also consistent with the client-centered philosophy of occupational therapy.[11] Further, Meichenbaum[8] has emphasized the importance of the child as a collaborator in the cognitive behavioral approach. He declared, "the children we treat have a great deal to tell us if we would only ask and then listen" (p. 96). Finally having children choose their own goals ensures ecological relevance, which promotes motivation, transfer and generalization. A daily activity log is provided to the child in advance of the goal-setting session. The log helps children reflect upon the activities that they do each day. At the beginning of the assessment phase, the COPM is used to ensure that the goals that will be focused on during intervention are child-chosen.

Dynamic Performance Analysis

The third key feature of CO-OP is dynamic performance analysis (DPA), a dynamic and iterative process of performance analysis, as it happens. (For a detailed discussion of DPA, please see Polatajko et al.[32]) DPA was developed in concert with the CO-OP approach to allow for continuous evaluation of performance and to structure the problem solving process. DPA begins during the first session and continues throughout the intervention. The purpose of DPA is to solve performance problems by identifying where performance breaks down, identifying possible solutions and testing them out in a trial and error fashion.

FIGURE 2. Session Structure: CO-OP Intervention Protocol

Prior to Therapy	**Preparation**
	1. Establish contact with parents
	2. Orient parents to Cognitive Orientation to daily Occupational Performance (CO-OP)
	3. Contract with parents to ensure resources and support
	4. Provide Daily Activity Log
	5. Check for child/parent and therapist prerequisites
Session 1	**Assessment**
	6. Review child's completed Daily Activity Log
	7. Administer Canadian Occupational Performance Measure (COPM) and identify three goals
	8. Baseline child's performance using the Performance Quality Rating Scale (PQRS)
Session 2	**Introduction of Global Cognitive Strategy**
	9. Introduce Global Cognitive Strategy: Goal-Plan-Do-Check
	1. Therapist introduces the puppet, Commander GoalPlan DoCheck
	2. Therapist maps Goal-Plan-Do-Check (GPDC) to a familiar task
	3. Child maps Goal-Plan-Do-Check to a familiar task
	4. Parents observe session and discuss application of GPDC at home
Sessions 3-11	**Acquisition**
	10. Conduct Dynamic Performance Analysis: Ongoing
	11. Facilitate the child's acquisition and application of the Global Cognitive Strategy: Goal-Plan-Do-Check
	12. Guide discovery of Domain Specific Strategies (DSS) and mediate their application to skill acquisition
	13. Apply Enabling Principles
	14. Teach parents/caregivers about Goal-Plan-Do-Check and applicable Domain Specific Strategies
	15. Educate parents/caregivers about their ongoing role in facilitating cognitive strategy use to promote skill acquisition
Session 12	**Consolidation**
	16. Re-administer COPM
	17. Re-administer baseline, using PQRS
	18. Probe child for generalization and transfer of Global and Domain Specific Strategies: GPDC and DSS
	19. Review and reinforce CO-OP approach, and cognitive strategy use with parents/caregivers

Dynamic performance analysis (DPA) is based on three assumptions regarding occupational performance: that *motivation* is a necessary prerequisite for successful performance; that an individual requires adequate *knowledge of a task* before he or she can successfully perform the task and that *occupational performance* is the result of the interaction of person, occupation, and environment.

- *Motivation:* In the motor learning literature, it has been well documented that an individual's motivation for participation in a task: (a) affects learning, (b) influences the acquisition of skill, task performance, and task persistence, (c) enhances the ability to deploy existing skills and knowledge, and (d) affects the willingness to continue when the task becomes exceedingly challenging.[33] If task motivation is not present, it will be very difficult, if not impossible, to carry out a valid performance analysis. In the CO-OP approach, motivation is ensured by the child-centred approach.
- *Task Knowledge:* Pressley, Borkowski and Schneider[5] have noted that a prerequisite to performance is an understanding of the task requirements. Brown, Pressley, Van Meter and Schuder[34] have provided evidence that task knowledge is integral to strategy development for performance. If at least rudimentary task knowledge is not present, it will also be difficult, if not impossible, to carry out a valid performance analysis. The study of the CO-OP approach by Mandich and colleagues[18] showed that task knowledge is often inadequate to support task performance in children with DCD, and that supplementing task knowledge results in improved performance.
- *Occupational Performance:* In the occupational therapy literature it is generally believed that occupational performance is the result of the interaction between the individual, the occupation and the environment.[11,20-28] Successful performance requires achieving a balance between the ability of the performer, and the supports and demands of the occupation and the environment. Competent occupational performance is considered to be the outcome of an interaction in which performer ability is in perfect balance with occupational and environmental supports and demands.[25,26] DPA focuses on identifying the specific imbalances that prevent successful performance. In CO-OP, a problem solving approach is used to identify the source of the imbalance and potential strategies for solving the imbalance. The study by Man-

dich and colleagues[18] showed that with children with DCD, strategy use can solve performance problems.

Cognitive Strategies

The fourth key feature of Cognitive Orientation to daily Occupational Performance (CO-OP) is cognitive strategy use. Cognitive strategies are cognitive operations over and above the processes that are a natural consequence of carrying out a task.[5] They are strategic thinking processes aimed at accomplishing goals. In CO-OP, two kinds of strategies are used: a global strategy and domain-specific strategies.

A *global strategy is* a general executive strategy that focuses on increasing metacognitive awareness and training the individual to self-monitor and self-evaluate.[35] The global strategy utilized in CO-OP, Goal-Plan-Do-Check, is a problem solving strategy adopted from the cognitive behavioral work of Meichenbaum.[8,35] It is represented in the form of the mnemonic, Goal-Plan-Do-Check, developed by Camp, Blom, Hebert, and VonDoorwick.[36] The global strategy provides a structure within which the therapist or child can talk through the problems encountered in task performance. When using the Goal-Plan-Do-Check framework, the child is taught to use the following line of self-talk:

GOAL:	What do I want to do?
PLAN:	How am I going to do it?
DO:	Do it! (carry out the plan)
CHECK:	How well did my plan work?

Meichenbaum[35] points out that each stage of the Goal-Plan-Do-Check strategy facilitate an aspect of metacognitive thinking. For instance, determining the GOAL requires self-interrogation, the PLAN requires the child to self-monitor, the DO demands self-observation, and the CHECK fuels self-evaluation and self-reinforcement. Using this global framework, the child learns to talk him or herself through the task, and to develop metacognitive problem solving skills.

The Goal-Plan-Do-Check strategy is a central feature of the CO-OP approach to treatment. It is taught to the child during the second intervention session, and reinforced throughout subsequent therapy sessions. It not only provides a global problem solving strategy for the child, but also provides a vehicle for discovering domain specific strategies. Some type of concrete reminder of this strategy, such as a puppet, is used throughout the intervention sessions. One example of this, Commander GoalPlanDoCheck is depicted in Figure 3.

Domain Specific Strategies are an array of specific cognitive strategies, which focus on facilitating or improving performance that are task, child, or situation specific. Mandich and her colleagues[18] identified eight domain specific strategies used in CO-OP: body position, task specification/modification, feeling the movement, verbal motor mnemonic, verbal rote script, verbal instruction, verbal self-instruction, and attention to doing.

During the CO-OP intervention, children are taught to talk themselves through occupational performance problems using the global cognitive strategy. This strategy is then used to frame the discovery of domain specific strategies that will enhance performance. The emphasis during intervention is on helping the child to see how he or she can

FIGURE 3. Commander GoalPlanDoCheck

GOAL

PLAN

DO

CHECK

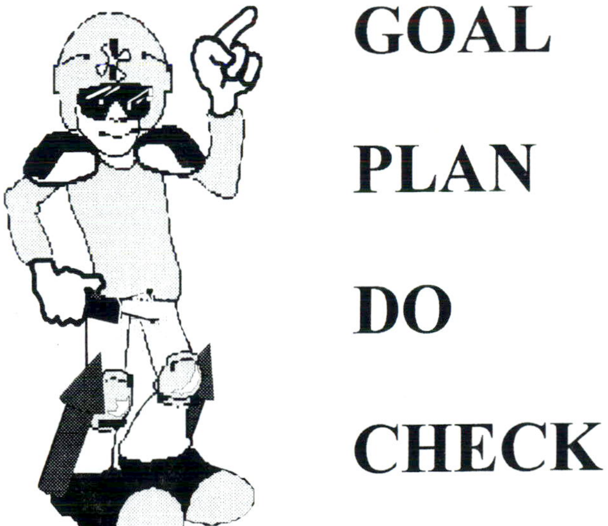

set goals, plan actions, talk him or herself through doing, and check outcomes. In other words, the focus is on metacognitive problem solving processes. The therapist helps the child to acquire occupational performance skills, by enabling the child's application of cognitive strategies to task performance.

Enabling Principles of CO-OP

A number of enabling principles have been developed for use in CO-OP to help the child learn to talk him/herself through occupational performance problems, use cognitive strategies, develop occupational skills and transfer and generalize learning. These have been drawn from general principles of learning, the literature on cognitive and mediation techniques, information about motor learning, and clinical experience with children with DCD.

Enabling principles are an integral part of the CO-OP therapeutic approach and are used throughout the therapeutic intervention. They are captured in 6 imperatives:

- *Make It Fun:* Experience with CO-OP indicates that therapists who are playful in their interactions with the children have the greatest success in getting children to use cognitive strategies and to improve occupational performance.
- *Promote Good Strategy Use:* Strategies form the bridge between abilities and skill acquisition. Pressley et al.[5] note that good strategy users have a number of characteristics in common. They suggest that effective use of cognitive strategies involves the coordination of several components including: sufficient task knowledge; a broad repertoire of strategies; and the realization that effort and strategy use affect performance. In CO-OP the therapist promotes good strategy use by: evaluating and supplementing the child's task knowledge as required, helping the child to develop a range of strategies, and guiding the child to see the connection between effort, strategy use and successful performance.
- *Frame It in Goal-Plan-Do-Check:* Throughout the intervention, the global strategy Goal-Plan-Do-Check provides the framework for solving performance problems. The therapist guides the child through the process of articulating the performance goal, developing a plan, carrying out the plan, and checking the effective-

ness of the plan. The focus is on teaching the child to use the global strategy to talk himself or herself through performance problems.

- *One Thing at a Time:* Children learn best when one thing is presented at a time. While the therapist may identify a number of issues that need to be addressed, it is important to keep the child focused on only one thing and not to place excessive attentional demands on the child.

- *Work Toward Independence:* The nature of the interaction between the therapist and child changes over the course of CO-OP intervention. During the initial phases, the therapist takes the lead role in modeling the application of the strategy. As the child becomes more competent in strategy use, the therapist slowly relinquishes the lead role so that the child can take the lead in solving performance problems. Throughout the intervention, the child is encouraged to apply the strategies in everyday situations. This is done by discussing opportunities for transfer and generalization with the child and parents at each treatment session and by assigning "homework" to be done between sessions.

- *Guided Discovery:* Children remember best when they discover something themselves. Therefore, in CO-OP the emphasis is on child discovery of strategies to support performance. Using a combination of Meichenbaum's[8,35] scaffolding techniques, and the mediational techniques of Feuerstein and colleagues[10,37,38] the therapist guides the child to discover the strategies that will help him or her perform the chosen activities. The process of guided discovery is illuminated by four catch phrases: "Ask, don't tell," "guide, don't adjust," "make it obvious," and "bridge beyond." The therapist also helps the child to develop and test out plans (as part of the Goal-Plan-Do-Check strategy) for achieving goals. The process of guided discovery is an iterative one and occurs throughout the therapy.

Parent/Caregiver Involvement

Parent involvement in the CO-OP approach is crucial to promote the child's ongoing skill acquisition, strategy use, and generalization and transfer of learning. The therapist can promote parental involvement by ensuring that parents learn about the salient features of CO-OP and the application of enabling principles. In this way the parent provides a critical link between the therapeutic setting and other environments. It has been recognized for some time now that involving parents in an intervention program promotes maintenance of learned behaviors and facilitates generalization and transfer.[39,40] Research indicates that students can achieve better outcomes at school when there is strong parental involvement.[41] Follow-up studies of behavior therapy have shown that children whose parents have been taught the behavioral techniques continue to improve and demonstrate transfer and generalization of improvement to areas that had not been specific treatment targets.[42]

In CO-OP, parents are required to observe Session Two, the session in which the global strategy is taught. They are then encouraged to help the child to practice applying the strategy before the next session. As well, parents are required to observe at least two additional treatment sessions and are strongly encouraged to participate in as many additional sessions as possible. Before each session begins, the therapist discusses, with the parent and child, the homework that was done. Examples are elicited of global and domain specific strategies that were used between sessions. Frequently parents use these opportunities to describe successes and discuss problems. At the end of each session, the strategies which emerged during treatment are reviewed and possible applications within the home and school environment are discussed.

CONCLUSION

CO-OP is a new approach to treatment for children with. In contrast to traditional approaches, CO-OP focuses directly on child-identified performance issues, and engages the child as an active problem solver and participant in the therapy process. Congruent with many contemporary ideas on skill development, CO-OP fosters the notion that performance is the result of the interaction between the child the environment and the occupation and that cognitive strategies can be used to drive performance. Use of the CO-OP approach, within a research paradigm, has provided evidence of the effectiveness of the approach with children with DCD. Further research is needed to investigate the use of CO-OP with other populations. This approach presents an alternative for therapists interested in a direct approach to the treatment of performance problems in children with DCD.

REFERENCES

1. Polatajko HJ. Developmental coordination disorder (DCD): Alias the clumsy child syndrome. In K Whitmore, H Hart, G Willems, (Eds.), *A Neurodevelopmental Approach to Specific Learning Disorders: The Clinical Nature of the Disorder* (pp. 119-133). London: MacKeith Press; 1999.

2. Mandich AD, Polatajko HJ, Macnab JJ, Miller LT. Treatment of children with developmental coordination disorder: What is the evidence? *Phys Occup Ther Ped.* 2001; 20(2/3), 51-68.

3. Gentile AM. The nature of skill acquisition: Therapeutic implications for children with movement disorders. In H Forssberg, H Hirschfeld, (Eds.), *Movement disorders in children* (pp. 31-40). New York: Karger; 1992.

4. Mathiowetz V, Haugen JB. Evaluation of motor behavior: Traditional and contemporary views. In CA Trombly, (Ed.), *Occupational therapy for physical dysfunction* (4th Ed.), (pp. 157-185). Baltimore: Williams and Wilkins; 1995.

5. Pressley M, Borkowski JG, Schneider W. Cognitive strategies: Good strategy users coordinate metacognition and knowledge. In R Vasta, (Ed.), *Annals of child development* (pp. 89-129). London, England: JAI Press; 1987.

6. Polatajko HJ, Macnab JJ, Anstett B, Malloy-Miller T, Murphy K, Noh S. A clinical trial of the process-oriented treatment approach for children with developmental co-ordination disorder. *Dev Med Child Neurol.* 1995; 37, 260-269.

7. Missiuna C, Mandich AD, Polatajko HJ, Malloy-Miller T. Cognitive Orientation to Daily Occupational Performance (CO-OP): Part I–Theoretical Foundations. *Phys Occup Ther Ped.* 2001; 20(2/3), 69-81.

8. Meichenbaum D. *Cognitive-behavior modification: An integrative approach.* New York: Plenum Press; 1977.

9. Feuerstein R, Haywood HC, Rand Y, Hoffman MB, Jensen MR. *Learning potential assessment device (L.P.A.D.) manual.* Jerusalem: Hadassah-Wizo-Canada Research Institute; 1986.

10. Haywood HC. A mediational teaching style. *The Thinking Teacher* 1987; 4, 1-7. John F. Kennedy Center for Research on Education and Human Development.

11. Canadian Association of Occupational Therapists. *Enabling Occupation: An occupational therapy perspective.* Ottawa, ON: CAOT Publications ACE; 1997.

12. Wilcox, A. L. Verbal self-guidance: An exploratory study with children with developmental coordination disorder. Unpublished master's thesis, The University of Western Ontario, London, ON Canada, 1994.

13. Wilcox A, Polatajko HJ. Verbal self-guidance as a treatment technique for children with developmental coordination disorder. (Abstract). *Can.J.Occup.Ther.* 1993; Supplement: 20-20.

14. Martini, R. Verbal self-guidance as an approach to the treatment of children with developmental coordination disorder: A systematic replication study. Unpublished master's thesis, The University of Western Ontario, London, ON Canada., 1994.

15. Martini R, Polatajko HJ. Verbal self-guidance in the treatment of children with developmental coordination disorder: A systematic replication study. (Abstract). *Can.J.Occup.Ther.* 1995;62:11.

16. Martini R, Polatajko HJ. Verbal self-guidance as a treatment approach for children with developmental coordination disorder: A systematic replication study. *Occup Ther J Res.* 1998; 18, 157-181.

17. Mandich, A. Cognitive Strategies and Motor Performance of Children with Developmental Coordination Disorder. Unpublished master's thesis, The University of Western Ontario, London, ON Canada, 1997.

18. Mandich AD, Polatajko HJ, Missiuna C, Miller LT. Cognitive strategies and motor performance in children with developmental coordination disorder. *Phys Occup Ther Ped.* 2001; 20(2/3), 125-143.

19. Polatajko HJ, Mandich AD, Miller LT, Macnab JJ. Cognitive Orientation to Daily Occupational Performance (CO-OP): Part II–The Evidence. *Phys Occup Ther Ped.* 2001; 20(2/3), 83-106.

20. Baum C. Client-centred practice in a changing health care system. In M Law, (Ed.), *Client-centred occupational therapy* (pp. 29-46). Thorofare, NJ: Slack Incorporated; 1998.

21. Christiansen CH, Baum CM. The occupational therapy context: Philosophy-principles-practice. In CH Christiansen, CM Baum, (Eds.), *Enabling function and well-being* (2nd Ed.), (pp. 26-45). Thorofare, NJ: Slack Incorporated; 1997.

22. Fisher AG. Uniting practice and theory in an occupational therapy framework–1998 Eleanor Clarke Slagle Lecture. *Am J Occup Ther.* 1998; 52, 509-521.

23. Kielhofner G. Introduction ot the model of human occupation. In G. Kielhofner, (Ed.), *A model of human occupation theory and application* (2nd Ed.), (pp. 1-8). Baltimore, MD: Williams & Wilkins; 1995.

24. Law M, Baptiste S, Carswell A, McColl MA, Polatajko HJ, Pollock N. *Canadian Occupational Performance Measure.* (3rd Ed.). Ottawa, ON: Canadian Association of Occupational Therapists; 1998.

25. Polatajko, H. J. 1992 Muriel driver lecture. Naming and framing occupational therapy: A lecture dedicated to the life of Nancy B. *Can J Occup Ther.* 1992; 59, 189-200.

26. Polatajko HJ. The treatment of children with mild motor difficulties in OT: What do we know now? (Abstract). *Proceedings of 11th International Congress of the World Federation of Occupational Therapists, London, England* 1994; 856-858.

27. Reed KL, Sanderson SR. *Concepts of occupational therapy.* (2nd Ed.). Baltimore, MD: Waverly Press, Inc; 1983.

28. Yerxa EJ. Dreams, dilemmas and decisions for occupational therapy practice in a new millennium: An American perspective. *Am J Occup Ther.* 1994; 48, 587-589.

29. Deatrick JA, Woodring BC, Tollefson TL. Children should be seen and heard: chronically ill children should have a voice in treatment decisions. *Health Progress.* 1990; 71, 76-79.

30. Lewis MA, Lewis CE. Consequences of empowering children to care for themselves. *Pediatrician.* 1990; 17, 63-67.

31. Pittman KP. Awakening child consumerism in health care. *Pediatric Nursing.* 1992; 18, 132-136.

32. Polatajko HJ, Mandich A, Martini R. Dynamic performance analysis: A framework for understanding occupational performance. *Am J Occup Ther.* 2000; 54, 65-72.

33. Dweck CS. Motivational processes affecting learning. *American Psychologist.* 1986; 41, 1040-1048.

34. Brown R, Pressley M, Van Meter P, Schuder T. A quasi-experimental validation of transactional strategies instruction with low-achieving second-grade readers. *Journal of Educational Psychology.* 1996; 88, 18-37.

35. Meichenbaum, D. Cognitive-behavior modification: Workshop presented at the Child and Parent Research Institute symposium. 1991.

36. Camp, B., Blom, G., Herbert, F., and Van Doorwick, W. Think aloud: A program for developing self-control in young aggressive boys. University of Colorado School of Medicine; 1976.

37. Feuerstein R, Rand Y, Haywood HC, Hoffman MB, Jensen MR. *Learning Potential Assessment Device (L.A.P.D.) manual.* Jerusalem: Hadassah-Wizo-Canada Research Institute; 1980.

38. Haywood HC. Bridging: A special technique of mediation. *The Thinking Teacher.* 1988; 4, 2-8. John F. Kennedy Center for Research on Education and Human Development.

39. Ross AO. *Psychological disorders of children: A behavioral approach to theory, research, and therapy.* New York, NY: McGraw-Hill Inc; 1974.

40. Ross AO. *Child behavior therapy: Principles, procedures, and empirical basis.* New York, NY: Wiley; 1981.

41. Willms JD. Indicators of mathematics achievement in Canadian elementary schools. In Statistics Canada and Human Resources Development Canada, (Ed.), *Growing up in Canada. National longitudinal survey of children and youth,* (pp. 69-82). Ottawa, ON Canada: Minister of Industry Catalogue No.89-550-MPE, no. 1; 1996.

42. Lovaas OI, Koegel R, Simmons JQ, Long JS. Some generalizations and follow-up measures on autistic children in behavior therapy. *Journal of Applied Behavioral Analysis.* 1973; 6, 131-166.

Cognitive Strategies
and Motor Performance in Children
with Developmental Coordination Disorder

Angela D. Mandich
Helene J. Polatajko
Cheryl Missiuna
Linda T. Miller

SUMMARY. Recently, researchers in occupational therapy have investigated the use of a cognitive or "top down" approach to improving the occupational performance of children with developmental coordination disorder. A cognitive approach is multifaceted in nature and one essen-

Angela D. Mandich, MSc, OT(C), is a doctoral candidate, School of Kinesiology, and Instructor, School of Occupational Therapy, The University of Western Ontario, London, Ontario, Canada. Helene J. Polatajko, PhD, OT(C), is Professor and Chair, Department of Occupational Therapy, Faculty of Medicine, University of Toronto, Toronto, Ontario, Canada. Cheryl Missiuna, PhD, OT(C), is Assistant Professor, School of Rehabilitation Science, and Co-Investigator, CanChild Centre for Childhood Disability Research, McMaster University, Hamilton, Ontario, Canada. Linda T. Miller, PhD, is Assistant Professor, School of Occupational Therapy, Faculty of Health Science, The University of Western Ontario. All of the authors are members of the Developmental Coordination Disorder Research Group.

Address correspondence to: Angela D. Mandich, School of Occupational Therapy, Faculty of Health Science, Elborn College, The University of Western Ontario, London, Ontario, Canada N6G 1H1 (E-mail: amandich@julian.uwo.ca).

This study was conducted as partial fulfillment of the requirements for the first author's degree of Master of Science in the School of Occupational Therapy, Faculty of Health Science, The University of Western Ontario.

[Haworth co-indexing entry note]: "Cognitive Strategies and Motor Performance in Children with Developmental Coordination Disorder." Mandich, Angela D. et al. Co-published simultaneously in *Physical & Occupational Therapy in Pediatrics* (The Haworth Press, Inc.) Vol. 20, No. 2/3, 2001, pp. 125-143; and: *Children with Developmental Coordination Disorder: Strategies for Success* (ed: Cheryl Missiuna) The Haworth Press, Inc., 2001, pp. 125-143. Single or multiple copies of this article are available for a fee from The Haworth Document Delivery Service [1-800-342-9678, 9:00 a.m. - 5:00 p.m. (EST). E-mail address: getinfo@haworthpressinc.com].

125

tial component of such an approach is the use of cognitive strategies. Although strategy use has a long history within the education and psychology literature, little discussion within the pediatric therapy literature has occurred. This paper reports the results of an in-depth videotape analysis of therapists using cognitive strategies during occupational therapy intervention. Eight domain specific strategies were identified and elucidated. This research will be beneficial to therapists who wish to incorporate a cognitive approach into their clinical practice. *[Article copies available for a fee from The Haworth Document Delivery Service: 1-800-342-9678. E-mail address: <getinfo@haworthpressinc.com> Website: <http://www.HaworthPress.com> © 2001 by The Haworth Press, Inc. All rights reserved.]*

KEYWORDS. DCD, intervention, cognitive strategies

There has been a call in the occupational therapy literature for the use of cognitive approaches to improve occupational performance in individuals with disabilities.[1,2,3] Toglia[3] has suggested that cognitive strategies can be used to enhance performance in adults with brain injury. Similarly, in the pediatric literature Goodgold-Edwards and Cermak[1] have suggested that strategies can be useful in teaching children new motor tasks.

The use of strategies to facilitate performance has had a long history in the cognitive theory literature.[4,5] It is only recently, however, that investigators in occupational therapy have explored the use of a cognitive approach for children with developmental coordination disorder.[6,7] An integral component of this cognitive or "top down" approach is the use of cognitive strategies. This shift to the use of a cognitive approach in occupational therapy parallels a paradigm shift in the literature pertaining to motor learning. Currently, there is a shift in motor learning theory suggesting that behavior is not hierarchically organized and arises from the interaction of many variables.[8,9] Mathowitz and Hagen[10] have described this shift in the occupational therapy literature suggesting its relevance to occupational performance.

LITERATURE REVIEW

For most children, skills of daily living such as cutting food, fastening zippers, handwriting, and rollerblading, are acquired incidentally.

However, a subgroup of children with apparently normal motor function struggle with the acquisition of such skills. These children have been described in the literature for decades, under a variety of labels.[11,12,13,14] In 1994, at the International Consensus Conference on Children and Clumsiness,[15] experts from around the world agreed that the term Developmental Coordination Disorder (DCD)[16] should be used when referring to children with such motor difficulties.[15] By definition, children with DCD demonstrate motor coordination difficulties that negatively impact on school performance and/or daily living.[16] Children with DCD are often referred to occupational therapy for a variety of performance deficits in particular, handwriting problems.[17]

Traditional occupational therapy intervention for these children has been based primarily on neuromaturational theories and treatment has focused on remediating underlying deficits in anticipation of a global improvement in motor performance.[17,18] More contemporary motor learning theories provide alternative ways of considering the problems of these children[19] and focus on the role that the context of the motor behavior plays in organizing the motor system for performance.[8,9] Dynamic systems theory proposes that behavior is self organized and emerges from various subsystems. These subsystems include "neuronal organization, muscle strength, joint structures and range of motion, motivational and arousal levels, support surface, and the task."[9]

Bouffard and Wall[19] and Henderson and Sugden[20] have argued that newer treatment approaches to DCD, based on more contemporary theories, need to be explored. Bouffard and Wall[19] have proposed the Problem Solving Approach that incorporates contemporary thinking from the motor learning, cognitive science, and cognitive psychology literatures. This approach focuses on cognitive and metacognitive processes and task variables in guiding motor behaviour. Henderson and Sugden[20] proposed the Cognitive Motor Approach, based on motor learning principles, to remediate deficits in children with motor difficulties. To date, these two approaches, theoretical in nature, have had limited clinical application.

The theoretical approaches described above parallel the investigation of a new cognitive approach. Recently, a group of occupational therapists[6,7,21,22,] have been developing and testing the use of a cognitive based approach to enable children with DCD to accomplish their occupational performance goals. This approach has its basis in cognitive behavioural theory[23] contemporary motor learning theory[10] and a philosophy of client-centredness.[6]

The approach, originally named verbal self-guidance (VSG),[6] uses a problem solving strategy, Goal-Plan-Do-Check (GPDC) described by Meichenbaum,[23,24] to enable children with DCD to learn three self-chosen motor skills. A series of 14 single case studies have been carried out to test this approach.[7,22] Results showed that, in all but one case, the GPDC strategy was able to be learned by children with DCD and was used to learn a variety of motor skills. In total, 13 of the 14 children with DCD, aged 7 to 12 years, learned to perform 39 motor tasks that the children had identified as difficult for them (i.e., cutting meat, throwing a ball, writing). These results, while in keeping with findings of the impact of a cognitive approach with other populations, provided the first evidence that a cognitive approach could be used successfully in the motor skill acquisition of children with a motor deficit.[a]

Wilcox[22] suggested that the possible variables related to improvement in occupational performance include the use of the GPDC strategy, the client-centered nature of the therapy, diagnostic task analysis, and parent involvement. However, Wilcox stated that a limitation of the study was that it "leaves the investigator without an understanding of which aspects of the intervention were most salient. A detailed analysis of videotapes would reveal the nature and pattern of mediational strategies that were precursors to the discovery, by the children, of the keys to occupational performance that resulted in their mastery" (p. 131).

Given the strong positive results of these early studies it is important to understand the salient features of this approach. The cognitive strategy literature[25,26,27] suggests that a single strategy (i.e., GPDC) may not be sufficient for the acquisition of skills and that executive or global strategies, such as GPDC, only lead to improved performance when other, domain-specific strategies are present.[26,27,28]

According to Pressley et al.[25] cognitive strategies are cognitive operations over and above the processes that are a natural consequence of carrying out a task. Strategies are both potentially conscious and controllable. The Good Strategy User Model (GSU)[26] suggests that effective strategy use involves the coordination of several components including: a broad repertoire of strategies, strategies that are global and some that are domain specific, the ability to know when and where to use these strategies, the realization that effort and strategy use effect performance, and that sufficient task knowledge is necessary. The types and usage of cognitive strategies during VSG intervention had not been previously investigated. Therefore, the objectives of this research study were:

1. To identify the cognitive strategies used during VSG intervention with children with DCD.
2. To classify the cognitive strategies observed during VSG intervention with children with DCD, using Pressley's Good Strategy User model.[26]

METHODS

This study employed behavioral observation to identify cognitive strategies used during VSG intervention sessions. Behavioral observation is used by many researchers in a spectrum of disciplines including sociology, psychology and special education.[29,30] Observation lends itself to the descriptive stage of research and is useful in producing hypotheses that can be used in further research.[31] Wilkinson[31] suggests that behavioral observation is particularly useful when researchers study the development of a new intervention or program.

Data Source

Data for this study were obtained from the videotaped intervention sessions of Wilcox and Martini.[17,22] According to Wilkinson,[31] videotape analysis allows for a level of detail and reliability not normally possible in a laboratory or formal observation in naturalistic settings. Observer bias can be readily checked by reviewing tapes with other observers and experts. The current study allowed a large quantity of videotaped data to be changed to a form that could be analyzed and collated.

All videotaped sessions occurred at The University of Western Ontario in the Department of Occupational Therapy. Wilcox's[22] study included ten children, and Martini's[7] study included four children.

All four children in Martini's[7] study were included in the present study. Four of the participants in Wilcox's[22] study were randomly chosen to be included in this study. Of the eight children selected, three were girls and five were boys.

Study Sample

The total sample consisted of 7,000 minutes of videotaped intervention sessions. First, ten, 10-minute segments were randomly chosen from each of the four children in Martini's study and from the four children randomly chosen from Wilcox's study. These 80 segments (800 minutes) of videotaped intervention were used to identify and classify strategies.

Development of Observational Coding Form

In this study an observational coding form was used for data collection. The observational coding form allowed for the systematic search for verbalizations of cognitive strategies over a 10-minute segment by recording the global task, transcribing the full dialogue of the therapist or child, recording the performance of the targeted behaviour, and recording whether the therapist or the child verbalized the strategy. The criterion for recording a strategy was that: (1) the strategy was discussed in words either by the therapist or the child; and, (2) immediate implementation of the stated strategy resulted in a change in observable motor behaviour. Change was considered to have occurred if the child performed the motor action.

Strategies that had been identified were classified. Proposed categories were examined and determined to meet the criteria of being exhaustive and mutually exclusive.[31,32,33] Although establishing behavioral taxonomies is extremely time consuming,[33] it ensures that codes are clear, complete, unambiguous and described in terms of observable characteristics.[31] There was no attempt to calculate frequency counts or averages for strategy use as summary statistics could lead to misinterpretations and inaccurate conclusions about strategy use and performance.[34]

Verification of Strategies

After development and refinement of the classification system, an independent observer was employed to verify the identification and classification of the strategies using new segments of videotape. The purpose was to ensure that the behavioural codes were mutually exclusive and exhaustive and that there were no strategies that fell into an undefined category.[31,32,33] Using procedures recommended by Martin and Pears,[35] interobserver agreement was first established. The primary investigator provided the observer with the data coding form. Following this, the investigator and the independent observer reviewed a total of 134 occurrences of strategies that had been recorded in the developmental phase. Interobserver agreement of 96% was established. Next, the independent observer and the primary investigator viewed 3, 10-minute segments of not previously viewed videotaped intervention sessions to ensure that the definitions were clear, and to establish interobserver agreement on videotaped data that had not been previously coded by either the independent observer or the primary investigator. Percentage agreement scores for these three segments were calculated at 94%, 92% and 96%, respectively. Next, 35, new 10-minute segments were randomly chosen from videotapes not used earlier to carry out an independent verification of the findings. Again, overt verbalizations that led to change in motor performance were recorded.

RESULTS

The findings of this study confirm the use of the global, executive strategy, Goal-Plan-Do-Check (GPDC) as reported by Wilcox and Martini.[7,22] In addition, several other components of the GSU Model described by Pressley et al.[26] were also evident. The GPDC strategy appeared to act as a global framework for invoking these other components of the GSU Model. Frequently, domain-specific strategies were required to enable the child to articulate the GOAL, or the PLAN, to DO the motor tasks or perform the CHECK. As well, it appeared that it was necessary to supplement task knowledge, a GSU component, in order for the children to be able to use the GPDC strategy. Table 1 summarizes the results of this study.

Higher Order Strategy Use: Goal-Plan-Do-Check

Observation showed that the global strategy Goal-Plan-Do-Check, formed the architecture for each intervention session. It was a vehicle

TABLE 1. Good Strategy User Components

A. Executive/Global Strategy

Goal Plan Do Check

B. Knowledge Base

Supplementing Task Knowledge

C. Strategy Use

Domain-Specific Strategies

1. Task Specification/Modification
2. Motor Mnemonic
3. Body Position
4. Feeling the Movement
5. Attention to Doing
6. Verbal Guidance
7. Verbal Self-Guidance
8. Verbal Rote Script

---

for the therapist and child to discover other strategies that assisted the child in achieving their occupational goals. This strategy occurred across all sessions and was used flexibly by both therapists.[22,7] In addition to being used in its entirety, various elements of the GPDC strategy were used in isolation. For example, the Plan was used in clarification and specification of the Goal. Also, in using the Check component, the child often evaluated whether the Plan was, in fact, effective. As a result of the Check, the child may have refined, or abandoned, the Plan. The Check component also served to confirm the effectiveness of the Plan. Through observation, each of the steps was able to be elaborated further than in previous work.

Goal: Determining the goal assisted in identifying the task for the sessions and providing a beginning focus for the session. Often, supplementing task knowledge was embedded in the goal. During the Goal stage, the motor behaviour was defined. At times, in the portions of the tapes observed the goal was very global such as "Our goal today is to print," and at alternate times the Goal was quite specific, such as "My goal is to print 3 capital B's." The goal was used to refine the expectations for the segment of the videotape observed. For example, in one case, the child stated "My goal is to cut cheese." The therapist further refined the goal to be "The goal is to cut the cheese all the same width."

Plan: The plan was often very iterative and elaborate. Typically, the plan required refinement and revision. When the child "got stuck" in an activity, the therapist would evoke the use of a domain-specific strategy to refine the plan. The therapist would analyze where the child was getting stuck. The child explored a variety of plans before arriving at one that worked for him/her. After execution of an ineffective plan, the child was required to revise his/her plan, generating alternative solutions to the plan. To illustrate, consider CT. While engaged in skipping, she stated "My plan is to jump." She attempted to jump, but continually got caught in the rope. Her plan required revision. Guided by the therapist, "When skipping you jump, but where do you jump?" the child responded after several attempts and revisions of the plan, "In the middle." When the therapist asked "Why?" the child responded, "because if you jump here you get caught." Then the therapist stated, "Let's try it, so your plan is to jump in the middle."

Do: The next step in this higher-order strategy was Do, the execution of the plan. Often descriptive verbalizations from the therapist accompanied the child's behaviour.

Check: The check component provided monitoring of the task. Check took many forms. Frequently taking the form of comparison, the children would compare examples of their own performance. Comparison also took the role of comparing performance with a model provided by the therapists or by a standard. At times, the results were self-evident. For example, during throwing a basketball, it was obvious whether the ball went in the hoop or not; or when jumping rope, if the rope got caught around the child's ankles, monitoring was self-evident. During other tasks, such as cutting tomatoes, achieving the same width for all slices required a greater precision of check. The Check component assisted in developing the criteria that acceptably defined successful task completion.

Additional Strategies

A number of strategies were observed that appeared to have a specific purpose in supporting the application of the Global Strategy during task performance. There appeared to be eight domain-specific strategies and also evidence of the therapist supplementing task knowledge. The observed behaviour for each strategy is defined in Table 2.

In the following section, the circumstances in which the strategy was used are presented, followed by a descriptive list of the behaviors that might be included under this category. Explicit scenarios de-

TABLE 2. Domain-Specific Strategies

Strategy	Observed Behaviour
Task Specification/ Modification	Any discussions regarding the specifics of the task or parts of the task, that facilitate motor performance. Modification of the task, or any action to change the task, or parts of the task, that facilitate motor performance.
Motor Mnemonic	Attachment of a label to the task or component of the task which evokes a mental image to guide motor performance.
Body Position	Verbalization of attention to, or shifting, of the body, whole or in part, relative to the task.
Feeling the Movement	Verbalization of attention to the feeling of the movement.
Attention to Doing	Verbalization to cue attending to the doing of the task.
Verbal Guidance	The therapist talks the child through the motor sequence.
Verbal Self-Guidance	The child talks him/her self through the motor sequence.
Verbal Rote Script	A rote pattern of words used to guide the motor sequence.

monstrating the use of each strategy and its motor performance outcome are also presented. Table 3 reflects a summary of the stage in the
problem-solving process that was mostly likely to elicited each strategy.

Supplementing Task Knowledge

Circumstances: It was clear from this videotape analysis that the
children frequently did not possess the basic knowledge necessary to
execute the motor task in question. In the segments observed, the
children appeared to lack an understanding of what the motoric task
requirements were. Supplemental task knowledge was provided to
assist the child in understanding the demands of the task. It was used
extensively by both therapists. It stood apart from the other domain-
specific strategies as this component was often a prerequisite to the
use of those strategies.

This component was observed to be used during a variety of videotape segments; some examples include developing an understanding
of aiming during hockey, understanding that when you print you start
at the left margin, and understanding that letters need to sit on the line.

Scenario: During the task of printing, SG did not always start at the
left margin. The printing would be started at various points on the line.
It was clear from the discussion that the child did not understand that
he needed to start all his printing at the red margin line. The therapist

TABLE 3. Strategies That Facilitated Use of the Global Strategy

CIRCUMSTANCE	STRATEGIES USED
When the child did not have enough information to specify the GOAL or PLAN	• Supplementing task knowledge • Task specification • Motor mnemonic
When the child could not DO the movement	• Task modification • Body position • Feeling the movement • Attention to doing
When the child could DO the movement but required verbal guidance to practice	• Verbal guidance • Verbal self-guidance • Verbal rote script

drew the child's focus to this by stating, "We start all our sentences at the red line." This additional knowledge of the task assisted the child in performing the task.

Task Specification/Modification

Circumstance: Both therapists again used this strategy across all segments observed. This strategy was used to develop the specific skill in question. When the child did not know the goal, or could not define the plan, this strategy was evoked.

Task specification was observed when the child did not understand the specifics of the goal and the plan; or when the child knew the plan, but could not perform the whole movement. The therapist would modify the task so the child could perform the modified task. Examples of this strategy were observed during the tasks of paper airplane making, learning to manipulate chopsticks, and learning to shoot a basketball.

Scenario: An example of task specification was observed with CT during skipping. CT had figured out that she needed to stand in the middle of the rope and jump, but she had trouble maintaining her body in the middle of the rope. The therapist said, "Let's put tape on the floor so you know where to stand." This specification assisted the child in monitoring where her body was relative to the rope. After the therapist placed the tape on the floor the child was able to maintain her body in the middle, using the tape as a guide.

Motor Mnemonic

Circumstance: Motor mnemonic was usually used when the child was specifying the goal or plan, or had difficulty remembering a movement pattern. It seemed that, by naming the movement in a way that had meaning for the child, motor performance improved. Both therapists used this strategy.

Scenario: When JW was learning to cut bread he could not cut even slices. The therapist suggested, "Let's notice what these fingers are doing." The child was able to discern, "I need to hold the bread," but could not figure out the position of the index finger. Through discussion, the child and the therapist identified his index finger as "Mr. Guard." Attaching this label to this particular behaviour elicited the desired behaviour in the child. The therapist then cued, "Remember Mr. Guard."

Body Position

Circumstance: This strategy was used by both therapists, across all segments observed, and concerned many positions including: holding the pencil properly, assuming a running stance, and sitting in an upright position while writing. Common to all the children was a difficulty with body positioning relative to the task at times. This strategy appeared to be used at times to adjust background positions, while at other times it became the focus of the activity. Once the child had an understanding of the task, the body position strategy facilitated the "doing" of the task.

Scenario: During the task of writing, when AB was focusing on the formation of the letter, the therapist would gently push his chair in to bring AB's body closer to the table and say, "Let's do this." Often using AB's own words, the therapist would guide him to an understanding of his body position relative to the task. The therapist questioned, "How close is your body to the table?" or "How should your back be in the chair?" The therapist reflected AB's response back to him; "Let's try writing when your back is against the back of the chair." The therapist had AB pull himself close to the table and identify the difference. Eventually AB discovered and verbalized, "I think my chair needs to be a bit closer to the table." In a final segment, AB was observed to sit down, but before beginning to write, pull his chair in, and correct his position without verbalizations.

Verbal Rote Script

Circumstance: This strategy was used to capture the essence of the movement in four or five clear, concise words that were meaningful to the child. It was observed to be used by both therapists during the segments of activities including, cutting cheese and karate. This sequence of words seemed to facilitate the execution of the movement. The therapist would recite the verbal script while the child performed the task. This strategy appeared to be used most often once the component parts of the skill had been mastered.

Scenario: During the activity of cutting cheese, JW was able to perform all the movements required with the use of the verbal rote script strategy. The therapist verbalized, "Hold, finger guard, down and push, hold, finger guard, down and push." This repeated sequence assisted JW in eliciting the movement.

Feeling the Movement

Circumstances: This strategy was used by both therapists, and was always initiated by the therapist. It was observed to be used only during the tasks of printing and writing. Once the child seemed to have a clear understanding of the task but was still unable to perform the movement, this strategy was evoked.

Scenario: AC was having difficulty learning the movement pattern, of the capital letter *B*. Frustrated by the difficulties she was having, AC stated, "I can't do them!" The therapist initiated the use of feeling the movement strategy. The therapist stated, "Well let's pretend, let's do it in the air; let's feel the bumps in the *B*." AC responded, "OK." The therapist continued, "Feel the bump, it splits in the middle." The therapist guided AC's finger through the formation of the letter and stated, "Now you make my finger move." AC stated, "I think I get it."

Attention to Doing

Circumstances: Attention to doing was used by both therapists. It was observed to be used effectively during the tasks of cutting tomatoes, learning to print, and nail painting. Generally, the children appeared to have some difficulty attending to the specifics of what they were doing. This strategy was evoked once the child had an understanding of the task requirements, but was getting stuck doing the task. Drawing the children's attention to what was required seemed to facilitate task performance.

Scenario: AC was having substantial difficulty cutting tomatoes. When the therapist stated, "Keep looking at what you are doing," AC was able to re-focus on the task and cut the tomato. During refinement of the behaviour of cutting tomatoes, the therapist would direct the child, "Let's notice the difference." "Look at which ones are the same." By attending to what the task required the child was able to compare and make appropriate accommodations that positively influenced motor performance.

Verbal Guidance

Circumstances: This strategy was always initiated by the therapist to elicit the desired motor pattern once the child could perform the movement. Both therapists used this strategy in all segments observed. During some motor tasks, tasks that have an arbitrary beginning and end, the therapist would talk the child through the sequence while the child was performing the movement. During other activities, the verbal guidance was provided before, or after, the execution of the desired behaviour.

Scenario: During the task of writing, AB was learning the formation of the letter *P.* AB was having difficulty orienting the letter to baseline. While he was completing the movement, the therapist stated, "First start at the top line and go all the way and touch the bottom line, then top of the line around and down."

Verbal Self-Guidance

Circumstance: This strategy was observed being used once the child had an understanding of the motor pattern required.

Scenario: During the task of writing, the therapist verbalized the sequence, "Down to this line then up to the top," while the child performed the movement. In a subsequent segment DS was observed quietly stating to himself, "Down, then up to the top."

DISCUSSION

The purpose of this study was to identify and classify the cognitive strategies observed during intervention with children with DCD. Results of this study identified several categories of strategies including a global strategy, domain-specific strategies, and the need for supplementing task knowledge. Further, the nature and application of the global strategy Goal-Plan-Do-Check was elucidated.

The findings of this study are consistent with the cognitive psychology literature[23,36,37] which indicates that cognition plays an active role in the acquisition of new skills. From behavioral observation of videotaped intervention sessions, it was noted that for children with DCD that cognitive strategies played a pivotal role in the learning of new motor behaviour during VSG intervention.

Observations of what transpired with regard to strategies used during the VSG intervention sessions were classified according to the Good Strategy User Model.[26] Consistent with this cognitive strategy perspective, several categories were observed. The synergistic interaction of global strategies, supplementing task knowledge and domain-specific strategies seemed to positively influence motor behavior. This study provides evidence that VSG is a complex intervention process. It seems that verbal self-guidance, as a strategy, is in fact only one strategy that is embedded among many.

Martini[7] and Wilcox[22] recognized that the use of VSG might precipitate the use of other cognitive strategies. In fact, Martini stated ". . . many factors involved in this approach remain unexplored. Exactly which aspects of this multifaceted approach are crucial for the clinician to comply with and which are not, still have to be determined" (p. 114).

From the results reported here, it would appear that domain-specific strategy use was an important part of VSG that was not previously recognized. Sternberg, Wagner, Williams, and Horvath[38] suggest that individuals possess a vast repertoire of tacit knowledge that is not readily accessible to description. Tacit knowledge is described as procedural. It may be that therapists use domain-specific strategies procedurally, without conscious realization of their usage.

The problem of identification of treatment variables has a long-standing history in the cognitive behaviour modification literature. Etscheidt[39] articulates that under the auspices of cognitive behaviour modification, different studies use different components, such as self-instruction training, reinforcement, and attributional training, yet do not clearly classify all components. This study is an initial attempt to identify parts of the VSG treatment that may influence motor behaviour. Whether, in fact, these strategies were integral to this intervention requires further study. However, if domain-specific strategies are integral, it becomes difficult to identify treatment variables, or study the efficacy of treatments, when the strategic techniques are present at a tacit level. It makes it difficult to teach other therapists an intervention technique if the treatment components are not well understood.

FUTURE DEVELOPMENT

The studies by Martini and Polatajko[21] and Wilcox[22] were limited by the small sample sizes and the nature of single case methodology.

Fawcett and Downs[39] argue that clinicians often attempt to determine the efficacy of treatment interventions before understanding of the components of the intervention and the underlying theoretical assumptions. This urgency to determine the effectiveness of intervention, before the key variables of the intervention are identified, needs to be tempered with descriptive research to identify those active variables. The results of this study provide an important beginning in understanding the components of VSG intervention; however further research is still required.

Videotape analysis is time consuming and costly; yet it is one way of recording and analyzing the complex interactions between the child and the therapist that may have influenced motor performance. A fundamental question remains as to whether cognitive strategies do affect performance. If our ultimate goal is to enhance occupational performance in children with DCD, then we must pursue investigations of VSG as it appears to be a promising approach.[b]

NOTES

a. The study that is described in detail in this paper was referred to as Study III in the paper by Polatajko, Mandich, Miller and Macnab, this volume.

b. As noted previously, since this study was completed, further research has been conducted by the Developmental Coordination Disorder Research Group and is reported in the series of three articles that present the development of a Cognitive Orientation to Daily Occupational Performance, this volume.

REFERENCES

1. Goodgold-Edwards SA, Cermak SA. Integrating motor control and motor learning concepts with neuropsychological perspectives on apraxia and developmental dyspraxia. *Am J Occup Ther* 1990;44:431-438.

2. Katz N. Occupational therapy's domain of concern: reconsidered. *Am J Occup Ther* 1985;39:518-524.

3. Toglia JP. Generalization of treatment: A multicontextual approach to cognitive perceptual impairment in adults with brain injury. *Am J Occup Ther* 1991;45:505-516.

4. Flavell JJ. Metacognition and cognitive monitoring: a new area of cognitive-developmental inquiry. *Am Psychol* 1979;34:906-911.

5. Flavell JH, Miller PH, Miller SA. *Cognitive development.* Englewood Cliffs, NJ: Simon & Schuster; 1993.

6. Wilcox AL, Polatajko HJ. Verbal self-guidance: a treatment technique for children with developmental coordination disorder. *Can J Occup Ther* [conference supplement] 1993;60:20.

7. Martini R. *Verbal self-guidance as an approach to the treatment of children with developmental coordination disorder: a systematic replication study* [Master's thesis]. London, ON: The University of Western Ontario; 1994.

8. Thelen E, Ulrich BD. Hidden skills: a dynamic systems analysis of treadmill stepping during the first year. *Society for Research in Child Development Monographs* 1991;56:1-98.

9. Ulrich BD. Dynamic systems theory and skill development in infants and children. In: Connolly KH, Forssberg H, eds. *Neurophysiology and neuropsychology of motor development.* London, UK: Mac Keith Press; 1997:319-345.

10. Mathiowetz V, Hagan JB. Motor behavior research: implications for therapeutic approaches to central nervous system dysfunction. *Am J Occup Ther* 1994;48: 733-745.

11. Gubbay S. The management of developmental apraxia. *Dev Med Child Neurol* 1978;20:643-646.

12. Henderson SE. The assessment of "clumsy" children: old and new approaches. *J Child Psychol Psychiatry* 1987;28:511-527.

13. Orton ST. *Reading, writing and speech problems in children.* New York, NY: WW Norton; 1937.

14. Walton JN, Ellis E, Court DM. Clumsy children: developmental apraxia and agnosia. *Brain* 1962;85;603-612.

15. Polatajko HP, Fox AM. *Final report on the conference children and clumsiness: a disability in search of definition.* London, ON: International Consensus Meeting; 1995.

16. American Psychiatric Association. Motor skills disorder 315.40. *Developmental Coordination Disorder. Diagnostic and statistical manual of mental disorders (DSM-IV).* 4th ed. Washington, DC: Author 1994:53-55.

17. Schaffer R, Law M, Polatajko H, Miller J. A study of children with learning disabilities and sensorimotor problems. *Phys Occup Ther Peds* 1989;9:101-117.

18. Ayres J. *Sensory integration and learning disorders.* Los Angeles, CA: Western Psychological Services; 1972.

19. Bouffard M, Wall AE. A problem solving approach to movement skill acquisition: implications for special populations. In: Reid G. ed. *Problems in movement control.* North-Holland: Elsevier Science; 1990.

20. Henderson SE, Sudden D. *The movement assessment battery for children.* London, UK: Psychological Corporation; 1992.

21. Martini R, Polatajko HJ. Verbal self-guidance as a treatment approach for children with developmental coordination disorder: a systematic replication study. *Occup Ther J Res.* In press 2000.

22. Wilcox A. *Verbal self-guidance: an exploratory study with children with developmental coordination disorder* [Master's Thesis]. London, ON: The University of Western Ontario; 1994.

23. Meichenbaum D. *Cognitive-behavior modification: an integrative approach.* New York, NY: Plenum Press; 1997.

24. Meichenbaum D. *Cognitive-behavior-modification.* One day workshop presented at the Child and Parent Resource Institute Symposium, London, ON; 1991.

25. Pressley M, Forrest-Pressley DL, Elliot-Faust D, Miller G. Children's use of cognitive strategies, how to teach strategies, and what to do if they can't be taught. In: Pressley M, Bainerd CJ. eds. *Cognitive Learning and Memory in Children.* New York, NY: Springer-Verlag; 1985:1-47.

26. Pressley M, Borkowski JG, Schneider W. Cognitive strategies: good strategy users coordinate metacognition and knowledge. In: Vasta R. ed. *Annals of child development.* Vol. 4. London, UK: JAI Press; 1987:89-129.

27. Sugrue B. A theory-based framework for assessing domain-specific problem-solving ability. *Educational measurement: issues and practice* 1995; Fall:29-35.

28. Tarver SG. Cognitive behavior modification, direct instruction and holistic approaches to the education of students with learning disabilities. *J Learn Disabil* 1986;19:368-375.

29. Etscheidt S. Reducing aggressive behavior and improving self-control: a cognitive-behavioral training program for behaviorally disordered adolescents. *Behav Disord* 1991;16:107-115.

30. Piaget J. *The child's conception of the world.* London, UK: Routledge & Kegan; 1951.

31. Wilkinson J. Direct observation. In: Breakwell GM, Hammond S, Fife-Schaw C. eds. *Research methods in psychology.* London, UK: Sage 1995:214-229.

32. Bakeman R, Gottman JM. *Observing interaction: an introduction to sequential analysis.* Cambridge, UK: Cambridge University;1986.

33. Observing behavior. In: Sackett GP. ed. *Theory and applications in mental retardation.* Vol. I. Baltimore, MD: University Park Press of Child Development 1978;4:89-129.

34. Siegler RS. The perils of averaging data over strategies: an example from children's addition. *J Exp Psychol Gen* 1987;116:250-264.

35. Martin G, Pears J. *Behavior modification: what it is and how to do it.* Englewood Cliffs, NJ: Prentice-Hall; 1992.

36. Luria AR. *The role of speech in the regulation of normal and abnormal behavior.* New York, NY: Liveright; 1961.

37. Vygotsky LS. *Thought and language* (Hanfmann E, Vakar G. trans.). Cambridge, MA: M.I.T. Press; 1962 [original work published 1934].

38. Sternberg RJ, Wagner RK, Williams WM, Horvath JA. Testing common sense. *Am Psychol* 1995;50:912-927.

39. Fawcett J, Downs FS. *The relationship of theory and research.* 2nd ed. Philadelphia, PA: FA Davis; 1992.

CLINICAL CONCERNS

Passport to Learning:
A Cognitive Intervention for Children
with Organizational Difficulties

Jeanie Leew

SUMMARY. Many children who are referred for therapy with school-related problems experience difficulty with impulsivity, task completion and the organization of information and ideas. School performance often improves when children learn to approach tasks systematically and to use cognitive strategies. In this paper, a short term, small group program is described that targets children's cognitive deficiencies and emphasizes a strategy-based, problem-solving approach to intervention. *[Article copies*

Jeanie Leew, BScOT, is an Occupational Therapist who works as a private practitioner with IDEAS: Integrated Developmental Educational and Assessment Services Incorporated.

Address correspondence to: Jeanie Leew, BScOT(C), 10325 Bonaventure Drive S.E. Calgary, Alberta, Canada T2J 7E4.

The author gratefully acknowledges Simon Kendall Design Ltd. for the creative drawings of Leo the Lion. The author sincerely thanks Cheryl Missiuna, for her helpful comments on earlier versions of this manuscript.

[Haworth co-indexing entry note]: "*Passport to Learning:* A Cognitive Intervention for Children with Organizational Difficulties." Leew, Jeanie. Co-published simultaneously in *Physical & Occupational Therapy in Pediatrics* (The Haworth Press, Inc.) Vol. 20, No. 2/3, 2001, pp. 145-159; and: *Children with Developmental Coordination Disorder: Strategies for Success* (ed: Cheryl Missiuna) The Haworth Press, Inc., 2001, pp. 145-159. Single or multiple copies of this article are available for a fee from The Haworth Document Delivery Service [1-800-342-9678, 9:00 a.m. - 5:00 p.m. (EST). E-mail address: getinfo@ haworthpressinc.com].

145

KEYWORDS. DCD, intervention, cognitive

For children between the ages of 6 and 12, school is a central and important part of their lives. Participation in school-related tasks and activities are critical to the development of academic, physical and social skills.[1] Children who are not coping well with the demands of the school environment may be referred to pediatric occupational therapists for intervention. Initial concerns that are expressed by teachers and parents most often include comments about the children's handwriting and written work. "Printing is illegible," "pencil grip is odd," "written work is all over the page," and "written products take a lot of effort" are representative of the types of remarks made on initial referral. Before beginning to intervene, most therapists take time to observe the child in the classroom and to interview teachers and parents further. At this point, additional, significant difficulties often become evident. Teachers and parents may comment that they have observed that the child "does not plan before starting tasks," "hurries through projects," "is careless," "is unaware when he has made a mistake," "does not attend to details," "has difficulty getting started," and "does not generalize what he learns from one day to the next." These and other similar types of concerns reflect a pattern of organizational difficulties that is typical of many children with learning disabilities (LD) attention deficit disorder (ADHD) and developmental coordination disorder (DCD).

Descriptions of handwriting approaches and programs abound in the literature.[2,3,4,5] Relatively less attention has been given, however, to the types of organizational difficulties that many children experience and that have a serious impact on school performance. Lack of organizational skills significantly diminishes the students ability to initiate tasks or complete work independently. Recent studies have shown that it is the attentional or organizational difficulties, when present in addition to poor motor skills, that contribute to poor outcomes in children with DCD.[6] In this paper, a short term program will be described that was developed to specifically address these types of difficulties with organization and task completion. The intervention, *Passport to Learning,* has been conducted as a ten-week, small group program that emphasizes a strategy-based, problem-solving approach to learning.

REVIEW OF THE LITERATURE

Passport to Learning developed from the theoretical principles and program guidelines that were originally outlined by Feuerstein and colleagues.[7,8] These theories were further described by Haywood and colleagues[9] and then applied with younger children in the Cognitive Curriculum for Young Children.[10] Finally, many of the theories have been brought together into the Cognitive Network Education Model (COGNET) that has been developed and researched by Greenberg.[11] In order to be succinct, each principle or technique that is used in *Passport to Learning* is described briefly below and a reference to its theoretical basis is provided from the literature. (To read more about the general application of mediational theories within occupational therapy in pediatrics, please see Missiuna, Malloy-Miller and Mandich.[12])

Mediated Learning Experience

The major underlying principle in *Passport to Learning* is that the therapist will become a mediator of a child's cognitive deficiencies and, in doing so, will help them to learn more efficiently. Feuerstein[7,8] believed that children's cognition could be modified, if a significant adult was willing to "mediate" the child's thought processes, effectively putting him or herself between the child and the activity. This mediated learning is accomplished by creating a safe, supportive, fun atmosphere where "content-free" activities are used to illustrate the need for specific thinking processes. School-based activities that also rely on the targeted thinking processes are then introduced. Specific strategies are taught, the selection of personal strategies is encouraged, discussed and then applied. In a mediational atmosphere, children realize that they are working as a team, they will not be put on the spot, and guidance will always be available.

Mediational Techniques

Haywood and colleagues[9] described some of the key techniques that a mediator will use when working with children. The major techniques used in *Passport to Learning* include:

a. *Process Questioning*–the therapist uses questions that help the child to focus on the process of thinking, not on the product;
b. *Bridging*–the therapist prompts the child to think of other situations or activities where the strategy that they have learned can be applied. This creates a "bridge" between the therapy session and other environments and helps to encourage generalization;
c. *Challenging*–the child is encouraged to focus on why the answer is correct and how he came up with the answer so that he will be able to do it correctly again;
d. *Describing*–the therapist encourages the child to use accurate and precise language when describing the activities, difficult points and possible solutions;
e. *Modeling*–the therapist thinks aloud, demonstrating the problem solving process, evaluation strategies and revision techniques;
f. *Reflection/Summarizing*–the therapist elaborates on the child's responses and actions and, using questions, helps the child review the things that contributed to or hindered success.

Cognitive Functions

Feuerstein believed that children's cognitive difficulties could be described by observing the way that they approached a task (input), seemed to think about it (elaboration) and responded to it (output). He developed a list of specific impairments in cognition at each phase[7] of a cognitive act. For pediatric therapists, it is more helpful to state the impairments in positive terms in order to highlight what the child should be able to do when performing daily tasks. The list of cognitive functions have been developed into an observational scale and can be seen in Table 1. The numbers represent a typical profile that shows the frequency with which most children in the program would demonstrate each cognitive function. Cognitive strategies that are introduced throughout the program are developed directly from the cognitive deficiencies observed in the children. So, for example, if children seem to be impulsive and do not attend to visual details before they begin a task, then the strategy of systematic searching and attention to detail might be taught.

Problem-Solving Framework

A step-by-step problem solving approach is used in every session and applied to every activity in *Passport to Learning*. The particular

TABLE 1. Passport to Learning–Cognitive Skills Observation Scale

5–always	4–frequently	3–usually	2–sometimes	1–never/rarely

Cognitive Function*	Rating **	Comments
1. Gathers clear and complete information	2	
2. Attention is focused	2	
3. Exhibits systematic exploration	1	
4. Uses labels to identify objects	3	
5. Uses spatial system of reference	2	
6. Is precise and accurate when needed	2	
7. Remembers and considers multiple sources of information	1	
8. Understands temporal concepts	3	
9. Recognizes and defines the problem	2	
10. Selects relevant vs. non relevant cues	1	
11. Spontaneously compares objects/events	2	
12. Projects learned relationships–bridges	2	
13. Forms mental picture of object/visualization	1	
14. Uses hypothetical thinking	2	
15. Thinks before answering, no trial and error	1	
16. Makes a plan to achieve goal	3	
17. Follows the plan to completion	1	
18. Perceives need for clear, precise responses	1	
19. Relating past to present experiences	1	
20. Restrains impulsive behavior	1	
21. Able to develop and generalize strategies	1	
22. Self checks finished product	2	
23. Able to remember/retrieve information	2	
24. Communication reflects awareness of the information perspective of the listener	1	

*Adapted from Feuerstein[7], Missiuna,[14] Meichenbaum[15]
**Typical ratings received by children who participate in this program

framework that is used is based on the four step program that was originally described by Camp and Basch[13] as a sequence of steps that were carried out by Ralph the Bear. Specific problem solving steps used in *Passport to Learning* are described later.

Mind-Mapping

Mind-mapping is a technique that involves graphic representation, organization and linking of ideas. A mind-map uses pictures, words and/or symbols to summarize and link strategies with activities or with their application. Mind-mapping is described in COGNET, a program that was designed to assist children who were considered to be high risk or underachievers to develop their thinking skills and improve their performance at school.[11]

DESCRIPTION OF PASSPORT TO LEARNING

This ten-week program has been offered on five separate occasions over the past two years. The age and number of the participants, and the setting, have varied; however, the group has usually been comprised of 6-8 children who have diagnoses of learning disabilities or attention deficit disorder. Children were usually between seven and ten years of age but the program has been used successfully with children up to 13 years of age who were mildly delayed in development. DCD is a diagnosis that is not often made but some of the children who have participated also show characteristics that are typical of children with DCD. Parent participation is not mandatory but is strongly encouraged. As described below, two of the sessions are specifically for the parents and attendance at these has been excellent.

Cognitive Deficiencies of the Children

In order to implement a cognitive approach of this type, it is believed to be important to ascertain the cognitive difficulties that the children are experiencing. Teachers will often describe that the child, "just can't seem to get organized by himself," "has great ideas but just can't seem to follow through," "does really well if I interpret the instructions and slow him down." The cognitive deficiencies outlined by Haywood[10] and Feuerstein[7] were used to develop an evaluation tool (see Table 1). This tool can be used during classroom observations, as part of an individual assessment or as a questionnaire that is completed by parents after the first parent session. Identifying each child's particular cognitive deficiencies is an important step in planning an individual program for each child.

Structure of the Program

Passport to Learning is a ten-week program that runs once per week for 90 minutes. This length of time seems to be optimal in order to complete the non-academic activities that target the cognitive deficiency and introduce the strategy and also to ensure sufficient time for academic application. Two of the sessions are parent sessions and eight of the sessions are conducted with the children. A teacher or parent helper is an asset, as long as they understand the importance of participants completing projects on their own. As described below, "homework" is assigned each week in order to encourage transfer of the skills that are taught to the school environment.

Description of the Parent Sessions

Two parent sessions are conducted as part of the ten-week course. Parent Session 1 is an orientation session. The goal of this session is to have parents understand, and begin to think about, how children learn. Parents are introduced to theoretical concepts of how children think and learn and to appreciate the difference between the process (problem-solving) and products (content) of learning activities. Feuerstein's theory of Cognitive Modifiability[7] is outlined with an emphasis upon the benefits of mediated learning experience. Cognitive functions as outlined by Feuerstein[7] and Haywood[10] are explained and described. The concept of becoming a mediator is discussed and specific mediational techniques such as process questioning and bridging are described.[9] The goals of the ten-week program are outlined and parents are introduced to the particular cognitive strategies that will need to be reinforced at home during each week. Leo the Lion's Problem-Solving Framework (described in the next section) is strongly emphasized so parents will go over the four steps involved in problem-solving whenever the opportunity arises.

Parent Session 2 is usually scheduled to occur at about week seven. Topics that were introduced during the orientation session are reviewed and explored in more detail. The key elements of a mediated learning experience are examined and any issues regarding use of the mediational techniques are discussed. "Homework assignments" are also discussed and parents are encouraged to share the applications and bridging opportunities that they have found to be most useful.

Description of the Student Sessions

In keeping with Feuerstein's[7] principles of building competence and intrinsic motivation, each session is designed to be fun and non-threatening. The therapist must be prepared to "think aloud" and demonstrate his/her own deficiencies and problem solving strategies. The therapist uses mediational techniques during every activity in order to get the children to become more aware of their thinking and learning processes.

Leo the Lion (see Figure 1) is an updated version of the Ralph the Bear series.[12] Leo and his tools are introduced during the first student session and are applied during every activity that the children do in the program. Leo outlines the four stages of problem solving as he asks himself: (Stage 1)"What is my problem?" (Stage 2) "How do I do it?" or "What is my plan?" (Stage 3) "Do it" (Stage 4) "How did I do?"

It is important that the therapist has a clear and complete lesson plan for each session but it is also necessary to ensure that there is sufficient flexibility that one can encourage discussion and exploration of ideas. Session one is described in detail in order to provide an illustra-

FIGURE 1. Leo the Lion and His Problem-Solving Steps

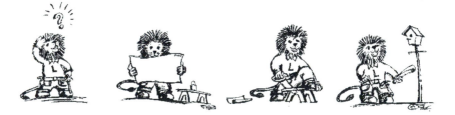

Reprinted with permission of Jeanie Leew.

tion of some of the key concepts and strategies that are involved in each session. The major concepts, activities, cognitive functions and strategies that are covered in each of the other seven student sessions are outlined in Table 2.

Student Session 1: Thinking About Thinking

Problem solving stage: What is my problem?
Key Concept: It is important to gather clear and complete information
Cognitive Strategies

- exploring systematically
- attending to visual details
- using labels to identify objects
- recognizing the need to be precise and accurate

Introduction: Why is this called *Passport to Learning?*
Introduce Leo the Lion (see Figure 1)

- he has a proper name (use of labels)
- look at him carefully (attend to visual details)
- he has all the right tools for the job (explore systematically)
- students need the right tools for each job (bridging)
- let's color his tools (recognize need to be precise and accurate)
- he is ready to work (introduce problem solving stages)

Orientation to Binders

- a binder is provided to each child with tabs for each week's activities
- a separate section is created for a vocabulary list (use of labels)

Non-Academic Activity: Construct a rotoglide plane

Children work on making the airplane. As they proceed, they are encouraged to talk aloud and cognitive strategies are identified that are helpful. In addition to the strategies that are the cognitive focus for the week, strategies may be discovered such as going slowly, finger tracing before drawing, making sure you have the

TABLE 2. Passport to Learning Session Outline

Week	Cognitive Focus	Activities "Content Free"	Occupational Application	Strategies*	Vocabulary	Bridging Homework**
1	Parent Introduction					
2	The problem solving approach Systematic exploration Comparing Restraining impulsivity	Looking at the Leo steps (see Figure 1) Coloring Leo Make a list of Leo's tools Rotoglide plane[16] Learn to draw activity	Identify personal tools needed for: school bag bathroom bag gym bag	Labeling Being precise Looking carefully Making a list	Strategy Example Model Precise	Complete school and bath personal tool kits Learn to draw Dart plane
3	Gathering clear and complete information Attention to relevant visual details Defining the problem	Where's Waldo[17] The Great Waldo Search[18] I Spy Fantasy Book[19]	Word searches Editing spelling errors Math signs Location activities: maps dictionary phone book	Looking at the model Searching systematically Verbal self guidance	Relevant detail Systematic	
4	Understanding spatial systems of reference N,S,E,W Communication reflects awareness of the information perspective of the listener	Orienteering/Compass Activities Describing locations Giving directions Looking at Constellations Map exploration	Geography Activities	Precise labeling	North, South, East, West	Practice giving and following directions using a reference system appropriately Risk Game
5	Understanding spatial systems of reference Right, Left Visual transport Part whole relationships Forming a mental picture of an idea	Room Mapping Blindman's Treasure Hunt Battleship Game Magazine Magic Explore architects' drawing	Map your school classroom Answer "where is" questions precisely Give clear verbal directions Story map techniques	Use a visual cue Talk aloud Use precision tools for drawing Go slowly	Beside, behind, Below, Above Left, Right Left of Right of Forward, Back. In relation to Relative to	Map your house Map your bedroom Map your school Map your closet, organize your closet

154

Week	Cognitive Focus	Activities non-academic	Occupational Application	Strategies	Vocabulary	Bridging Homework
6	Make a plan to achieve a goal Anticipating difficulty	Stained glass windows constructed with tissue paper Look at the finished product and create written instructions Highlight the trickiest step	Outline the steps in a division question Highlight the trickiest step:	Number the steps Use clear, concise instructions Label materials Use proper terms	Anticipate Plan Tricky Concise Efficient	Cooking activities
7	Parent Session					
8	Evaluating	Creating evaluation scales for previous projects that have been completed	Printing evaluation FBS3 SCALE Formation, baseline Size, speed, space	Look carefully	Edit Evaluate Inspect	Ask teachers for evaluation criteria Ask mom how she evaluates a babysitter
9	Recognizing the need to use a plan Selecting appropriate strategies to complete a project. Anticipating difficulties Analyzing errors Revising	Doll chain Beaded Gekko		(Review strategies that have already been learned)	Revise Adjust	
10	Summarizing/ Celebrating	Mind map of the program	Student led activity	Review		

*Students create "Personal Strategy Cards"
**Success Steps Worksheets are used for all home projects to encourage generalization of the problem-solving framework and the strategies

155

appropriate tools for the job, attending to the model and self talk. Children record strategies on strategy cue cards. Vocabulary cue cards are also begun.

Academic Application

Children are asked to make a list of items that you need to have in your pencil case at school and a list of items (tools) they will need each week for this group.

Conclusion

A verbal and/or written summary of the session is used to capture the main concepts and ensure that they are clear. A "mind map" can be used to summarize key points and strategies. Sometimes the children verbally summarize a "rule" of the day. A bridging discussion is then held to encourage the children to think of other opportunities for application of the cognitive strategy. For example, systematic search is a good strategy to use with dictionaries, telephone books, crosswords and word searches. Attending to visual details is helpful in geography and science tasks. Children are then assigned "homework"; in this case, to make another type of paper airplane at home. At the beginning of the subsequent session, homework is reviewed and the strategies of the previous week are reinforced before any new strategies are introduced.

Parent Support

Parents are asked to have the children explain what they learned in the session. Parents are provided with written information about the specific cognitive focus and strategies that have been introduced and a list of ideas for activities that will encourage strategy use. Parents are asked to discuss other activities that require precision and systematic exploration and to encourage the child to use accurate labels. Finally, instructions for the homework assignment are provided and a "Success Steps" sheet is attached. This sheet requires the child to record their homework in writing under these headings: The Problem/Goal, The Plan, The Tricky Parts, How to Do It, How to Strategies, and Check it Over. The steps that led to success in the homework are reviewed at the beginning of the next session.

Additional Considerations

Depending upon the age of the participants and the size of the group, different techniques can be used to make sessions more interesting and understandable. With some groups, Leo has been a hand puppet. In other cases, children have been encouraged to draw bubbles above the cartoon pictures and to write down what Leo is "thinking." Non-academic activities can also vary with the age and interest of the group. It is important to always select activities that are highly dependent upon the cognitive function that is being taught. For example, when trying to elicit examples of where else it is really important to be precise, a junior high group of girls came up with "nail painting." We used this as our application activity in the next session as it was very meaningful to the students. The girls were able to generate numerous strategies that would contribute to precise execution.

Another important consideration is to create an atmosphere in which sessions are long enough and children are allowed to take as much time as they need to successfully complete tasks. In *Passport to Learning,* students are often encouraged to take a second try at the same project once they have evaluated their work and realized what strategies they need to focus on. Comparing first attempts to second attempts is both enlightening and rewarding. It is imperative that students experience success and that they link the strategies to a product that they are proud of and that they completed on their own. Employing new cognitive strategies such as planning, searching systematically and executing precisely is very time consuming at first and it is critical that students not be rushed and provided with the answer too quickly. Many of these children have word retrieval problems and are slow to complete tasks: one thing that makes these sessions different from school is that they know they will have time to answer and time to finish the project independently.

A final comment must be made about the impact of this program on children's self-esteem and perceptions of their competence. By about the fourth week of the program, it becomes apparent that the children are gaining confidence in their own abilities. The early emphasis on information gathering strategies and problem solving steps enables them to approach and complete tasks independently. The focus on precision strategies leads to success and genuine pride in finished projects.

CONCLUSIONS

The program described in this paper is a cognitive approach to intervention that has been used with small groups of children who were experiencing organizational difficulties and problems with task completion. Beginning from a theoretical assumption that some of the children's cognitive processes are deficient, one therapist has developed a ten-week program that emphasizes problem-solving and the teaching of cognitive strategies. It is hard for children to talk about their thinking unless they are provided with a language and vocabulary to describe their thinking processes. In *Passport to Learning*, children learn the vocabulary that they need and learn to talk out loud about their thinking. This program has been successful in helping children to take control of their own learning and in identifying changes that they need to make to improve their performance at school. The approach is practical and is applied to tasks that are difficult for the child on a daily basis. Children have been observed to transfer and generalize the strategies to the classroom when they ask teachers to provide a model, to outline steps for an activity or to state clearly criteria for evaluation. Parents have been found to be able to learn and employ the mediational techniques and the problem solving questions which also encourages generalization.

In the future, it is hoped that this type of program might be attempted within the regular classroom, or in a resource room. Participation of the teacher has been found to facilitate the application and bridging of strategies to academic material. Further development of the program, and systematic research, is also needed.

REFERENCES

1. King GA. School-based practice. In GA King, (Ed.), Special issue on school based practice. *Phys Occup Ther Pediatr.* 1999; 19(2), 1-3.

2. Bonney MA. Understanding and assessing handwriting difficulty: Perspectives from the literature. *Aust Occup Ther J.* 1992; 39, 7-15.

3. Harris SJ, Livesey DJ. Improving handwriting through kinesthetic sensitivity practice. *Austr Occup Ther J.* 1992; 39, 23-27.

4. Lockhart J, Law M. The effectiveness of a multisensory writing program for improving cursive writing ability in children with sensorimotor difficulties. *Can J Occup Ther.* 1994; 61, 206-214.

5. Oliver CE. A sensorimotor program for improving writing readiness skills in elementary-age children. *Am J Occup Ther.* 1990; 44, 111-116.

6. Kadesjo B, Gillberg C. Attention deficits and clumsiness in 7-year-old Swedish children. *Dev Med Child Neur.* 1998; 40, 796-804.

7. Feuerstein R, Rand Y, Hoffman MB, Miller R. *Instrumental Enrichment: An intervention program for cognitive modifiability.* Baltimore MD: University Park Press. 1980.

8. Feuerstein R, Rand Y, Hoffman MB. *The Dynamic Assessment of Retarded Performers: The Learning Potential Assessment Device, Theory, Instruments and Techniques.* Baltimore MD: University Park Press. 1979.

9. Haywood HC. A mediational teaching style. *Thinking Teacher.* 1987; 4,1-6

10. Haywood HC, Brooks P, Burns S. *Bright Start Cognitive Curriculum for Young Children.* Waterdown, MA: Charlesbridge Publishing. 1992.

11. Greenberg K *Cognitive enrichment advantage teacher handbook.* Chicago, IL: Skylight Training. 2000.

12. Missiuna C, Malloy-Miller T, Mandich A. Mediational techniques: Origins and application to occupational therapy in pediatrics. *Can J Occup Ther.* 1998; 65, 202-209.

13. Camp BW, Bash MA. *Think aloud.* Champaign, IL: Research Press. 1981.

14. Missiuna C. *Dynamic assessment of preschool children with special needs: Comparison of mediation and instruction.* Unpublished master's thesis. Calgary, AB: University of Calgary, 1986.

15. Meichenbaum D. *Cognitive-behaviour modification.* Workshop presented at the Child and Parent Resource Institute symposium. London, ON. 1991.

16. Francis N, Bradford J. *Paper airplanes and other super flyers (rotoglide).* Toronto, ON: Kids Can Press Ltd. 1996.

17. Handford M. *The great Waldo search.* Boston, MD: Little Brown and Company. 1989.

18. Handford M. *Where's Waldo?* Toronto, ON: Grolier Limited. 1991.

19. Marzolla J, Wick W. *I Spy Fantasy: A book of picture riddles.* New York, NY: Scholastic Inc. 1994.

Index